Acid Reflux Cookbook

Relieve GERD, LPR and Heartburn with 100 Delicious Recipes and Easy-to-Follow Advices | + 60 Day Meal Plan

Evelyn Rivers

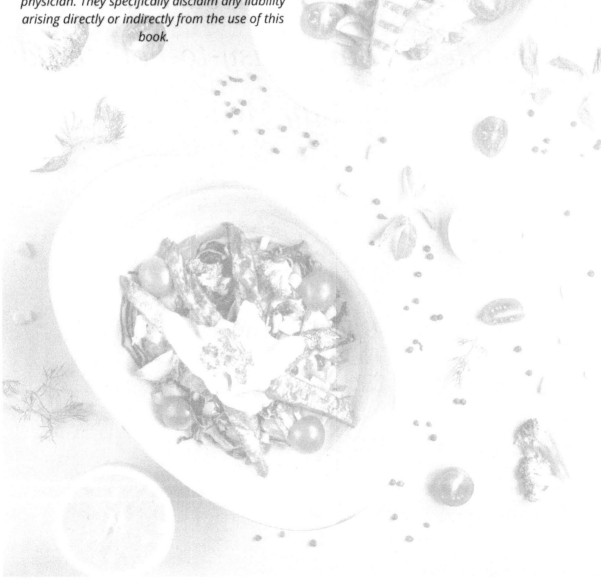

SCAN THE QR CODE

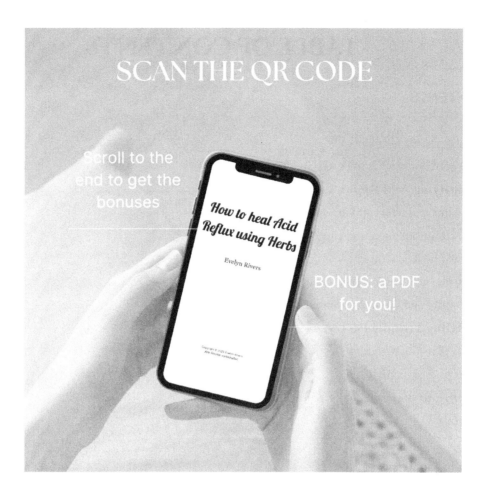

Scroll to the end to get the bonuses

How to heal Acid Reflux using Herbs

Evelyn Rivers

BONUS: a PDF for you!

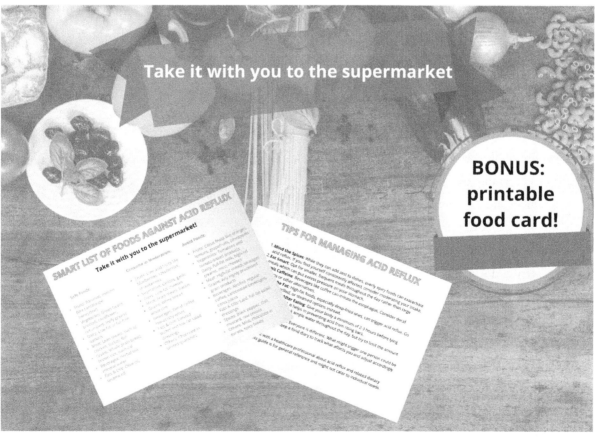

Take it with you to the supermarket

BONUS: printable food card!

TABLE OF CONTENTS

Introduction

Acid reflux: a daily battle for many

Acid reflux is a constant daily battle for numerous people all over the world, not simply a one-time post-meal discomfort. This condition, which is frequently seen as a minor inconvenience, can seriously interrupt a person's day-to-day activities, making ordinary tasks like eating, sleeping down, or even laughing triggers for pain and discomfort.

The Invisible Adversary

Fundamentally, acid reflux, also known as gastroesophageal reflux disease (GERD), is a condition that develops when stomach acid or bile runs upward into the esophagus, resulting in the burning sensation that is generally referred to as heartburn. Although it can seem simple, the subtleties of its impact go well beyond the physical. Many people's symptoms don't merely involve a chest burn. They may feel anything, including a persistent cough, trouble swallowing, or a choking sensation.

The Daily Struggle

Consider arranging your day to accommodate your symptoms and attempting to anticipate when they will next manifest. Food, clothing (avoid wearing tight belts or waistbands), and even social activities can all be influenced by the fear of an unplanned episode of reflux. Casual outings are turned into workouts in anticipation to make sure you won't be too far from help if it's needed.

Mealtimes, which ought to be enjoyable and relaxing times, can instead become stressful. Even eating, which should excite and nourish us, may turn into a minefield where the wrong food decision can cause hours of misery.

Even at night, it is not always a haven of peace. Many people who suffer from severe reflux fear falling asleep flat because the acid will rise uninvitedly, disrupting their sleep.

The Emotional and Mental Toll

It can be emotionally taxing to deal with the unpredictable nature of acid reflux on a regular basis. Feelings of loneliness, irritability, and even despair might result from a constant need to stay vigilant and modify one's lifestyle to accommodate the symptoms. Many people with the condition discover that they must avoid specific activities they once loved or refrain from social situations where food is involved.

The ongoing research, attempting each at-home or over-the-counter remedy, looking for a break, and the recurrent disappointment when something doesn't work can also leave one mentally exhausted.

A Journey, Not a Destination

Despite the constant struggles, it's critical to acknowledge acid reflux for what it is: a treatable ailment. One's quality of life can be regained with the appropriate information, dietary decisions, and occasionally medical assistance. Even though it might not be a quick win, many people have fought and won this battle before.

With the help of this book, you should be better equipped to deal with acid reflux. You may transform this everyday struggle into a successful campaign for comfort and well-being via knowledge, planning, and the appropriate techniques.

Navigating the cookbook: what to expect and how to use

Welcome to a gourmet trip that will not only entice your taste buds but also calm your stomach and esophagus. This book is more than just another cookbook; it's a handcrafted manual meant to change the way you view food. Every page of this book is committed to bringing comfort, understanding, and enjoyment, with a focus on helping those who have acid reflux. In order to make the most of this cookbook, let's first discuss its organization before getting into the recipes and advice.

Structure of the Cookbook

1. **Foundational Knowledge**: The first sections are devoted to describing acid reflux, its causes, and how nutrition affects it. Not only are the recipes important, but also the 'why' behind them.

2. **Food Lists**: We have lists of foods that are "safe" and "potential triggers." These lists serve as a quick reference for your food shopping and are supported by research and useful ideas.

3. **Diverse Recipes**: You'll find a wealth of dishes created just for people who suffer with acid reflux, from breakfasts that help you start the day without discomfort to meals that guarantee restful nights.

4. **Lifestyle Tips**: This book examines planning, eating habits, and other aspects of acid reflux that go beyond food.

5. **Interactive Sections**: This cookbook can now serve as a customized acid reflux diary thanks to the spaces we've provided for you to take notes, monitor your symptoms, and evaluate your progress.

How to Use This Cookbook

1. **Start with Understanding**: Before jumping into the recipes, take some time to read the initial chapters. Grasping the science and reasoning behind acid reflux can empower your dietary choices.

2. **Personalize Your Experience**: Everyone's body is unique. What makes someone feel uneasy could be safe for someone else. As you try several recipes, make notes on how they make you feel and alter and modify as you go.

3. **Plan Ahead**: Your culinary journey will be seamless thanks to the meal planning and preparation portions. Spending some time in advance preparing can prevent you from eating meals that could cause symptoms.

4. **Engage with the bookenjoy**: Utilize the interactive features. Follow your symptoms, make a list of your favourite dishes, and mark the ones you wish to try.

5. **Experiment and Enjoy**: Don't be scared to play around with flavour and substitute combinations. The recipes are only suggestions, and your palette is different. Find out what suits you the most.

6. **Seek Community**: It's possible to cook together. Talk about your experiences with friends, family, and online communities. You'll discover that lots of people are on like journeys and can offer advice, suggestions, or just a listening ear.

A Lifelong Companion

Remember that this book is meant to develop with you as you go through it. Your understanding of your body, your connection with food, and even the degree of your acid reflux can change over time. Allow this cookbook to be a versatile resource that responds to your needs and brings solace and relief at each point of your journey. Here's to many more heartburn-free meals in the future as you enjoy the recipes and treasure your moments of discovery!

Chapter 1: Demystifying Acid Reflux

The science behind acid reflux and its symptoms

Heartburn, also known as acid reflux, is a condition that lasts longer than the brief discomfort that follows a heavy meal. It is a sophisticated physiological event that has its roots in human anatomy and bodily chemical processes. We need to learn more about the science governing our digestive system and what occurs when things go wrong in order to fully comprehend acid reflux. Join me as we set off on this scientific adventure.

Digestion: A Delicate Ballet

After being consumed, food is meticulously broken down into smaller components for our body to utilise during digestion. It begins in the mouth, travels through the esophagus, and finally enters the stomach, where enzymes and acids are crucial in breaking down the meal.

- **Esophagus**: A muscular tube that carries food from the mouth to the stomach.
- **Stomac:** The Lower Esophageal Sphincter (LES), which separates the esophagus and stomach, is a vital organ. The LES functions as a one-way valve, permitting food to enter the stomach while obstructing the flow of stomach contents, including acid, back into the esophagus.

The Unwanted Backflow

Acid reflux occurs when the LES doesn't function correctly. Instead of remaining tightly closed, it might relax inappropriately or weaken, allowing the stomach acid to flow back (or 'reflux') into the esophagus. This backflow is what causes the characteristic burning sensation.

Symptoms: Beyond Just Heartburn

While heartburn – a burning sensation in the chest – is the most recognized symptom of acid reflux, the condition can manifest in various ways:

1. **Regurgitation**: A sour or bitter-tasting acid moving up into the throat or mouth.
2. **Dysphagia**: A sensation of a lump in the throat, leading to difficulty or discomfort in swallowing.
3. **Chest Pain**: Sometimes mistaken for heart-related conditions, this pain can be sharp and burning.
4. **Dry Cough**: A persistent cough that isn't related to colds or other respiratory issues.
5. **Hoarseness**: A change in voice quality and persistent sore throat.
6. **Bloating**: A feeling of fullness or swelling in the stomach.
7. **Hiccuping and Burping**: Especially if persistent and occurring shortly after meals.
8. **Nausea**: An urge to vomit, which can sometimes lead to actual vomiting.

Factors That Contribute to LES Dysfunction

Multiple factors can lead the LES to malfunction:

1. **Certain Foods and Drinks**: Ingredients like caffeine, chocolate, alcohol, peppermint, and fatty foods can relax the LES.
2. **Medications**: Some medicines, including aspirin and certain muscle relaxants, can cause the LES to relax.
3. **Hiatal Hernia**: A condition where the upper part of the stomach bulges into the chest through an opening in the diaphragm, affecting LES function.
4. **Smoking**: Chemicals in tobacco can weaken the LES.
5. **Pregnancy**: Increased pressure in the abdomen during pregnancy can cause reflux.
6. **Delayed Stomach Emptying**: Also known as gastroparesis, this condition can increase the likelihood of reflux.

Why Acid Hurts

The stomach's lining has a protective mucous barrier against the strong acid it produces. The esophagus doesn't. When acid refluxes into the esophagus, it irritates the sensitive lining, causing the symptoms we associate with acid reflux.

Understanding Leads to Better Management

While acid reflux can seem a mere inconvenience for some, recognizing its root causes and the science behind its symptoms provides a foundational understanding that can empower sufferers to manage it better. By aligning this knowledge with dietary and lifestyle choices, it becomes possible to navigate the challenges of acid reflux and significantly improve one's quality of life.

Unraveling the common causes and triggers

At the heart of managing acid reflux lies the understanding of its causes and triggers. While the physiological mechanism of acid reflux is rooted in the dysfunction of the LES, it's crucial to recognize the myriad factors that can instigate or exacerbate this malfunction. By unraveling these causes, we empower ourselves to take proactive measures to reduce and manage acid reflux symptoms.

Distinguishing Between Causes and Triggers

Before we delve deeper, it's essential to differentiate between causes and triggers:

- **Causes** refer to the underlying conditions or habits that predispose one to acid reflux. They set the stage for the condition.
- **Triggers** are specific events or substances that can provoke an episode of acid reflux in someone already predisposed to the condition.

Common Causes of Acid Reflux

1. **Hiatal Hernia**: This occurs when the upper part of the stomach pushes through the diaphragm into the chest cavity. It can weaken the LES, making acid reflux more likely.

2. **Obesity**: Excess fat, especially in the abdominal area, can increase pressure on the stomach, pushing acid into the esophagus.

3. **Pregnancy**: Hormonal changes combined with the growing fetus can lead to increased acid reflux.

4. **Connective Tissue Disorders**: Conditions like scleroderma can affect the muscles of the esophagus, leading to acid reflux.

5. **Delayed Stomach Emptying**: Conditions like gastroparesis, where the stomach doesn't empty properly, can cause acid to accumulate and then reflux.

6. **Smoking**: Chemicals in tobacco can cause the LES to relax, making reflux more likely.

Common Triggers for Acid Reflux Episodes

1. **Dietary Choices**:

- **Fatty and Fried Foods**: These can slow down digestion and relax the LES.
- **Tomato-based Foods**: Such as pasta sauces, pizzas, and soups.
- **Citrus Fruits and Juices**: Like oranges, lemons, and grapefruits.
- **Chocolate**: Contains caffeine and other compounds that can trigger reflux.
- **Mint**: Especially in large quantities.
- **Caffeinated Beverages**: Coffee and certain teas.
- **Alcoholic Drinks**: Especially when consumed in excess.
- **Spicy Foods**: Though the reaction varies from person to person.
- **Onions and Garlic**: Especially when raw.

2. **Medications**: Some drugs, including aspirin, certain anti-inflammatory drugs, some blood pressure medications, and certain muscle relaxants, can induce acid reflux.

3. **Large Meals**: Overeating can increase stomach pressure, leading to reflux, especially when lying down shortly after eating.

4. **Carbonated Drinks**: The bubbles can expand inside the stomach, increasing pressure.

5. **Lifestyle Habits**: Lying down immediately after eating, rigorous physical activity right after a meal, or even wearing extremely tight clothing can induce episodes of acid reflux.

Listening to Your Body

While lists of common causes and triggers provide a helpful starting point, it's essential to understand that everyone is unique. A food or activity that triggers reflux in one person might be completely fine for another.

To truly navigate the challenges of acid reflux, it's crucial to become attuned to your body's signals. Keeping a symptom journal, noting what you ate or did before each reflux episode, can help identify personal triggers and pave the way for tailored management strategies.

A Proactive Approach

Understanding the common causes and triggers is the first step. The next is integrating this knowledge into daily life, making informed dietary and lifestyle choices to minimize the risk of acid reflux episodes. Armed with knowledge and proactive strategies, living with acid reflux becomes not a daunting challenge but a manageable condition.

Chapter 2: Red Flag Foods

Ah, food! It's the center of so many of our life's moments, isn't it? From the family dinners to the solo late-night snacks, it's the stuff that memories are made of. I mean, who can forget grandma's legendary mashed potatoes or that summer where all you ate was pineapple and somehow didn't turn into one?

But when it comes to our uninvited guest (you remember, acid reflux from our previous chat?), certain foods are like the uber-luxe VIP pass that guarantees its appearance. Picture this: a flashy neon sign that screams "Welcome!" with fireworks on the side. Yeah, some foods are just like that for our stomachs.

Red Flag Foods: The Real Culprits

Let's go on a bit of a culinary journey, shall we? Now, I know we've all got our guilty pleasures. For me, it's those extra cheesy, slightly burned on the edge, pepperoni pizzas. I swear I could eat them for breakfast, lunch, and dinner. But here's the deal: some of these tasty treasures come with a hidden cost, and it's not just the extra time on the treadmill.

Ever gone on a date, where right from the start, you knew it wasn't going to work out? Maybe they had a weird laugh, or they just couldn't stop talking about their pet iguana. Well, some foods and our stomachs are on those exact kind of dates. Let's chat about a few of them.

Chocolates. Yep, I'm starting with the heartbreaker. While they're oh-so-delicious, they contain caffeine and other stimulants which can cause our esophagus to relax, allowing stomach acid to splash up. It's like opening the floodgates at a concert. Pandemonium!

Spicy Foods. Now, I love a good kick in my food. But here's the deal: these fiery delights can be super triggering. They're like the frenemies of the food world. They lure you in with their tantalizing tastes and then – bam! – heartburn central.

Fried and Fatty Foods. Ah, the siren song of crispy fries and rich, creamy sauces. These slow down digestion, keeping the food in the stomach longer. Think of it as the overstay of the food world. You had a great party, everyone had fun, but now they just won't leave, and things are starting to get uncomfortable.

Alcohol and Carbonated Drinks. Imagine this: you're throwing a party, and there's always that one guest who amps up the volume, making everyone louder and rowdier. That's what these drinks do. They increase stomach acid and can be quite the instigators.

1. Fatty and Fried Foods

Why They're Troublesome: Fats slow down the stomach-emptying process, resulting in prolonged acid production. Moreover, the added pressure from a stomach filled with fatty foods can force the LES to open, allowing acid to creep up.

Alternatives: Opt for lean cuts of meat, bake instead of frying, and reduce the use of oils and butter in cooking.

2. Citrus Fruits and Juices

Why They're Troublesome: Their inherent acidic nature can irritate an already inflamed esophagus.

Alternatives: Go for non-citrus fruits such as melons, bananas, or apples. If you crave citrus, consider diluting citrus juices with water or consuming them in smaller quantities.

3. Tomato-Based Products

Why They're Troublesome: Similar to citrus, tomatoes and their products are naturally acidic.

Alternatives: Opt for cream-based sauces or pesto. For dishes like salads, use non-acidic dressings or simple olive oil and herbs.

4. Spicy Foods

Why They're Troublesome: Capsaicin, the compound that makes foods spicy, can irritate the esophagus.

Alternatives: Use mild herbs and spices such as basil, oregano, or turmeric to add flavor without the heat.

5. Mint

Why They're Troublesome: While mint can soothe many stomach issues, it might relax the LES, exacerbating reflux in some individuals.

Alternatives: Try ginger as a calming alternative; it can soothe the stomach without triggering reflux.

6. Chocolate

Why They're Troublesome: Chocolate contains caffeine, fat, and other compounds that can trigger reflux.

Alternatives: If you're a chocolate lover, consider dark chocolate in moderation, as it generally has less fat and caffeine than milk chocolate.

7. Coffee and Caffeinated Drinks

Why They're Troublesome: Caffeine can relax the LES, making reflux more likely.

Alternatives: Opt for decaffeinated varieties or herbal teas like chamomile, which are less likely to cause reflux.

8. Alcoholic Beverages

Why They're Troublesome: Alcohol can relax the LES and increase stomach acid production.

Alternatives: If you do consume alcohol, do so in moderation. Choose drinks that are lower in alcohol content, and avoid mixing with acidic or carbonated beverages.

9. Onions and Garlic

Why They're Troublesome: They can be irritating to some individuals, triggering reflux.

Alternatives: Use herbs or milder flavors to season food. If you must use onions, cooking them thoroughly can reduce their potential to cause discomfort.

10. Carbonated Beverages

Why They're Troublesome: The carbonation can increase stomach pressure, forcing acid into the esophagus.

Alternatives: Flat water, herbal teas, or diluted non-citrus juices are safer choices.

Tuning Into Your Body's Signals

It's important to emphasize that while the above foods are common culprits, not everyone with acid reflux will react to all of them in the same way. It's crucial to monitor your body's reactions, and maybe even keep a food diary, to determine your personal triggers.

Understanding the 'why' behind their effects

The realm of food and digestion, while wondrous in its design, is a complex web of interactions, with each food playing a particular role in the story of our gastrointestinal health. The stomach, central to our discussion, functions optimally in a delicate balance. However, introduce acid reflux into the equation, and suddenly, we find ourselves navigating a tricky terrain, trying to discern friend from foe.

Diving into the specifics, let's first talk about the heart of our digestive process: the stomach. It's an organ designed for efficiency, producing hydrochloric acid, which is pivotal in breaking down the food we consume. However, there's a catch. This acid, as essential as it is, can sometimes become a troublemaker, especially when it decides to venture upward, into the esophagus.

You might wonder, what spurs this rebellious streak in stomach acid? The answer lies partly in the foods we consume. Certain culprits, like caffeine, rich chocolates, and fatty delights, tend to meddle with the function of the Lower Esophageal Sphincter (LES). The LES acts as a sentinel, ensuring the stomach contents stay where they belong. When it's relaxed or weakened by these foods, the probability of acid reflux increases.

Moreover, the narrative becomes more intricate when we consider the dynamics of digestion. Fatty foods, delicious as they may be, have a propensity to linger in the stomach, delaying the process of gastric emptying. This delay subsequently exerts more pressure on the LES, amplifying the risk of acid intrusion into the esophagus.

Spicy foods bring their own set of challenges. Capsaicin, the compound responsible for the heat in chili peppers, doesn't just tickle our taste buds. It can irritate the esophageal lining, and in some instances, stimulate the stomach to produce even more acid, thereby heightening the risk of reflux episodes.

The story doesn't end there. Carbonated beverages, popular among many, contain carbon dioxide that forms effervescence. This fizz, when consumed, translates into increased gas and pressure in the stomach. It's akin to adding more passengers to an already packed elevator; the increased pressure can compromise the LES's function.

Even foods with natural benefits can sometimes contribute to reflux concerns. Onions and garlic, staples in many culinary dishes, can occasionally be problematic, especially when consumed raw. They have the potential to stimulate greater acid production in the stomach. Additionally, being fermentable, they might lead to increased gas generation.

Lastly, a word on caffeine: while it's the revered elixir for waking up our minds, it has a lesser-known side. It can relax the LES, making the barrier between the stomach and esophagus more permeable to acid intrusion.

Strategies to identify and sidestep potential triggers

Navigating the world of acid reflux can sometimes feel like tiptoeing through a maze with surprises at every corner. Some of these surprises are pleasant, while others? Not so much. The good news is, with the right strategies, you can uncover your unique acid reflux triggers and learn to sidestep them gracefully.
Let's dive in together, shall we?

Crafting a Food Diary: Imagine having a personal detective by your side, detailing your food choices and their aftermath. That's what a food diary is like! Jot down your meals, and if something feels off afterward, make a note. Over time, this detective work helps unveil patterns, spotlighting foods that might not be your best pals.

The Art of Elimination: Think of this as a culinary experiment. For a while, step away from foods infamous for sparking acid reflux. Once the coast feels clear, bring them back into the fold, one at a time. It's like introducing old friends to a new group and seeing who gets along. If a particular food causes a scene (or in this case, a flare-up), you've found a potential trigger.

Being Wise with Portions: Ever attended a buffet and felt the urge to sample everything, only to regret it later? In the world of acid reflux, moderation is key. Instead of three grand feasts, consider smaller, more frequent meals. It's kinder to your LES and helps you figure out which foods, especially in larger helpings, might be the culprits.

Savoring Every Bite: There's a joy in savoring food, feeling its texture, and relishing its taste. Mindful eating isn't just about enjoyment, though. By being present, you can pick up early signs of discomfort, allowing you to identify and sidestep triggers before they wreak havoc.

The pH Litmus Test: Remember those pH strips from science class? They're not just for experiments. Testing the pH of unfamiliar foods gives you a hint about their acid reflux potential. It's like having insider information, helping you make wiser dietary choices.

Keeping an Ear to the Ground: The world of acid reflux research is ever-evolving. Keeping abreast of the latest studies and findings ensures you're always in the know, allowing you to adapt your strategies accordingly.

Teaming Up with Experts: Consider teaming up with a gastroenterologist or nutritionist. They bring a wealth of knowledge to the table, offering deeper insights, suggesting specific tests, and tailoring strategies to fit you perfectly.

Tuning into the Acid Reflux Community: There's comfort in shared experiences. Engaging with others on their acid reflux journey can be enlightening. While everyone's triggers might differ, there's always something to learn, a new tip to try, or a potential trigger you might not have thought of.

Chapter 3: The Reflux-Friendly Pantry

Ingredients that play nice with reflux

Living with acid reflux doesn't mean you have to compromise on flavorful, nutritious foods. While some ingredients might exacerbate symptoms, many others are gentle on the stomach and can be a delightful addition to your meals. This chapter offers a guide on how to stock your pantry, refrigerator, and freezer with reflux-friendly ingredients, ensuring you're always prepared for a tasty, symptom-free meal.

1. The Power of Whole Grains

The Basics: Grains such as oatmeal, brown rice, quinoa, and whole grain bread and pasta.

The Benefits: These grains are not only packed with nutrients but are also less likely to trigger reflux. Their fiber content aids in digestion and promotes a healthy gut.

Shopping Tips: Look for products labeled as "whole grain" or "100% whole wheat." Be wary of products that say "multi-grain" as they might not be entirely made of whole grains.

2. Lean Proteins: Your Best Friends

The Basics: Poultry (skinless), fish, lean cuts of beef, tofu, and legumes.

The Benefits: Lean proteins are essential for muscle repair and growth and can be easier on the stomach compared to their fatty counterparts.

Shopping Tips: Opt for grass-fed, organic, or wild-caught options when available and financially feasible.

3. Fresh Veggies: A Bounty of Benefits

The Basics: Green beans, peas, broccoli, carrots, and leafy greens.

The Benefits: Not only are these vegetables nutrient-rich, but they also tend to be low in acid, making them gentle on the esophagus.

Shopping Tips: Fresh or frozen are both great options. Avoid canned versions that might be preserved in acidic solutions.

4. Rooting for Root Vegetables

The Basics: Potatoes, sweet potatoes, beets, and parsnips.

The Benefits: Root vegetables are starchy, filling, and can act as a neutral base in many dishes, reducing the overall acidity of a meal.

Shopping Tips: Opt for organic when possible, especially if you prefer to consume them with the skin on.

5. Fruits that Soothe

The Basics: Melons (like cantaloupe and honeydew), bananas, pears, and apples.

The Benefits: While many fruits are acidic, these particular choices are less likely to trigger reflux symptoms and can provide a sweet relief in meals.

Shopping Tips: Buy fresh or frozen. If opting for canned versions, ensure they are stored in natural juice without added citric acid.

6. Dairy Alternatives

The Basics: Almond milk, oat milk, and other non-dairy alternatives.

The Benefits: For some, dairy can be a reflux trigger. These alternatives can offer a creamy texture without the associated symptoms.

Shopping Tips: Look for unsweetened versions to avoid added sugars. Ensure they are fortified with calcium and vitamin D for added health benefits.

7. Healthy Fats in Moderation

The Basics: Avocado, olive oil, and flaxseeds.

The Benefits: While fats can be a trigger for some, healthy fats consumed in moderation can be beneficial for overall health and satiety.

Shopping Tips: Choose cold-pressed, extra-virgin olive oil for the most health benefits. When selecting avocados, ensure they yield slightly to gentle pressure for optimal ripeness.

8. The Magic of Herbs and Spices

The Basics: Ginger, fennel, parsley, and chamomile.

The Benefits: These herbs and spices can be soothing for the stomach and provide flavor without the heat of spicier counterparts.

Shopping Tips: Fresh is often best, but dried versions can also be used. For ginger, consider keeping some in the freezer; it grates easier and lasts longer.

Conclusion: Building a Reflux-Friendly Kitchen

With the right ingredients on hand, living with acid reflux becomes less about avoiding triggers and more about enjoying a diverse range of delicious, nutritious foods. Investing time in understanding and stocking up on reflux-friendly ingredients can transform your daily meals from a potential source of discomfort to a joyous culinary adventure. Remember, the journey to a comfortable gut starts with what's on your plate. Armed with this guide, you're well on your way to a happier, symptom-free relationship with food.

Health benefits of these ingredients

Let's talk about the remarkable benefits of the ingredients we've chosen for this cookbook. Sure, our primary goal is to ease acid reflux symptoms, but the goodness of these ingredients doesn't stop there. They're packed with nutrients that promote holistic health, making them excellent choices for anyone aiming for overall well-being.

When we say "whole grains," we're not just talking about good gut health. Think oatmeal, quinoa, and other fiber-packed grains. They're fantastic for digestion, but did you know they're also champions for heart health? And if you're keen on stabilizing those blood sugar levels, whole grains are your best friends.

Now, when it comes to lean proteins - the likes of poultry, fish, tofu, and legumes - they're more than just the building blocks of life. Apart from their role in muscle maintenance and growth, they can also rev up your metabolism and help keep those hunger pangs at bay.

Ever think of fresh veggies like broccoli, carrots, and peas as nature's multivitamin? Because they are! Packed with essential vitamins and minerals, these veggies not only fuel numerous body functions but are also armed with antioxidants to fight off oxidative stress. And let's not forget they're low-cal wonders.

And speaking of vegetables, root veggies are nutritional treasures. Beyond providing that comforting, earthy taste, foods like potatoes and sweet potatoes are loaded with vitamins and complex carbs that keep you energized throughout the day.

Fruits, on the other hand, are nature's sweet treats, offering more than just delightful flavors. They hydrate, provide essential vitamins and minerals, and even support heart health.

If you're considering dairy alternatives like almond milk or oat milk, you're in for a treat. They're often fortified with nutrients essential for bone health, and their plant-based nature means zero cholesterol.

Now, don't even get me started on healthy fats. Avocado, olive oil, flaxseeds - they nourish your body and mind. Essential for brain function, glowing skin, lustrous hair, and even hormone production, these fats are truly multifunctional.

Lastly, the little giants in our food world: herbs and spices. These tiny additions, from ginger to chamomile, are brimming with health benefits. They can fight inflammation, soothe your digestive tract, and boost your immune system with their antioxidant properties.

Integrating them into your daily meals

Let's talk about making these reflux-friendly ingredients a seamless part of your daily meals. You might think it's a daunting task, but trust me, it's easier and more delicious than you'd imagine. Here's a quick guide on how to effortlessly and tastefully incorporate them into your meals.

Imagine waking up and treating yourself to a slice of whole grain toast instead of that white bread. Now, jazz it up with some almond butter and banana slices – what a wonderful, heartburn-free way to start your day! And if you're an oatmeal fan, why not try overnight oats with almond milk? Toss in some chia seeds, vanilla, and when morning comes, top it off with apples and a hint of cinnamon.

Come lunchtime, think about that refreshing quinoa salad. Picture cooked quinoa tossed with veggies like cucumber and cherry tomatoes, some grilled chicken, olive oil, and finished with parsley. Or maybe you fancy some lettuce wraps? Use them to bundle up tofu, avocado, and carrots, and oh, that ginger-soy dipping sauce on the side is a game-changer.

Snacking is where it gets even more interesting. Ever thought of dipping whole-grain crackers into freshly made guacamole? Or perhaps a smoothie made with oat milk and honeydew melon sounds more like your jam? And yes, throw in some flaxseeds for that extra health kick.

Dinner could be a beautiful ensemble of roasted root veggies like sweet potatoes and parsnips, dressed in olive oil and rosemary. And to make it wholesome, how about some baked fish on the side? Or, if you're craving something more oriental, a chicken stir-fry loaded with greens, served over brown rice might hit the spot.

Desserts? Of course, we've got you! A heartwarming oat and apple crumble or perhaps a refreshing melon salad drizzled with chamomile-infused syrup will ensure your sweet tooth is satisfied without unsettling your stomach.

And when it comes to drinks, imagine winding down with a cup of soothing chamomile tea or kickstarting your day with a turmeric latte made with almond milk.

Now, a few golden tips to keep in mind:

- Set aside some time for meal planning. Trust me, it keeps things smooth and keeps those unhelpful temptations at bay.
- Don't shy away from experimenting in the kitchen. Sometimes, the best recipes come from a bit of adventurous tweaking.
- Oh, and batch cooking? A lifesaver. Make large quantities of staples like quinoa or rice and use them as a base for different meals.
- And when you're out shopping, take a moment to glance at the labels. Opting for products that align with our reflux-friendly journey makes a world of difference.
- Lastly, surround yourself with inspiration. Follow those blogs, join communities, and maybe invest in a cookbook or two. Keep that passion for food alive!

Chapter 4: Breakfast

Breakfast, often celebrated as the most vital meal of the day, plays a pivotal role in setting the tone for the hours that lie ahead. It serves as the day's opening act, effectively breaking the fast of the night and infusing our bodies and minds with the essential fuel needed to embark on the day's adventures.

However, for those grappling with the discomfort of acid reflux, this crucial meal can sometimes evoke a sense of unease. Many traditional breakfast foods have the potential to trigger discomfort and disrupt the tranquility of your morning.

In this dedicated "Breakfast Recipes" chapter, our mission is to transform your morning menu into a source of delight and nourishment. Within these pages, you'll discover a collection of recipes thoughtfully curated to be not only gentle on the stomach but also an absolute delight for your senses. Here, the soft glow of the morning sun meets a culinary symphony, promising a harmonious blend of taste and tranquility.

These breakfast creations are not just about satisfying hunger; they are crafted with your comfort in mind. Each recipe is designed to minimize the risk of acid reflux discomfort, allowing you to savor every bite without worry. With these dishes, you can welcome the day with a smile, knowing that you've embarked on a journey where delicious flavors and peaceful mornings coexist in perfect harmony.

Recipes

Whole Grain Pancakes

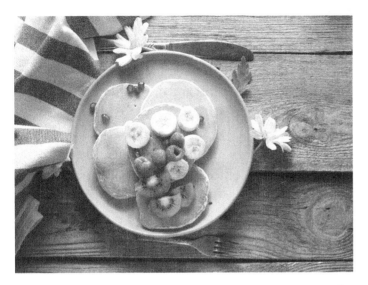

Preparation Time: 10 minutes | Cooking Time: 20 minutes | Portion Size: 4 servings (about 12 pancakes)

Ingredients:
- 1 1/2 cups whole wheat flour (or other whole grain flour)
- 2 tsp baking powder
- 1/4 tsp baking soda
- A pinch of salt
- 2 tbsp pure maple syrup
- 1 1/2 cups unsweetened almond milk (or another non-dairy milk)
- 1 large egg (or flax egg for a vegan alternative)
- 2 tbsp coconut oil, melted (plus extra for the pan)
- 1 tsp vanilla extract
- Optional toppings: Fresh berries, a drizzle of honey, or almond butter

Instructions:

In a large mixing bowl, whisk together the whole wheat flour, baking powder, baking soda, and salt.

In another bowl, combine the maple syrup, almond milk, egg, melted coconut oil, and vanilla extract. Mix until smooth.

Pour the wet ingredients into the dry ingredients and stir just until combined. Be careful not to overmix.

Heat a non-stick skillet or griddle over medium heat and lightly grease with a bit of coconut oil.

Pour 1/4 cup batter onto the skillet for each pancake. Cook until bubbles form on the surface and the edges look set, about 2-3 minutes. Flip and cook for an additional 2-3 minutes or until golden brown and cooked through.

Repeat with the remaining batter, adding more coconut oil to the skillet as needed.

Serve warm with your choice of toppings.

Nutritional Data: Calories: 280 | Total Fat: 10g | Saturated Fat: 7g | Cholesterol: 50mg | Sodium: 280mg | Total Carbohydrates: 40g | Dietary Fiber: 5g | Sugars: 8g | Protein: 7g

Note: Nutritional data are per 1 serving. They can vary based on the specific brands and amounts of ingredients used. It's always a good idea to double-check with a nutrition calculator if exact accuracy is essential.

Turmeric Oatmeal

Time to Prepare: 5 minutes | Time to Cook: 15 minutes | Portion Size: 2 serves

Ingredients:
- rolled oats, 1 cup
- 2 cups almond milk (or any non-dairy milk) that hasn't been sweetened
- Ground turmeric, 1 teaspoon
- Ground cinnamon, 1/2 tsp.
- One tablespoon of maple syrup, or to taste
- A pinch of black pepper (helps with turmeric absorption)
- Freshly sliced fruits (like banana or apple) for topping
- A sprinkle of chia seeds or flaxseeds for added nutrition (optional)
- A small handful of crushed nuts (like almonds or walnuts) for crunch (optional)

Instructions:

In a medium saucepan, bring the almond milk to a low boil. Add in the rolled oats and reduce the heat, allowing the mixture to simmer. As the oats start to absorb the milk and become tender (about 5 minutes in), stir in the ground turmeric, cinnamon, and black pepper. Continue to cook, frequently stirring, until the oatmeal reaches your desired consistency, roughly 10-12 minutes. Once cooked, remove from the heat and stir in the maple syrup.
Serve warm in bowls. Top with freshly sliced fruits, chia or flaxseeds, and crushed nuts, if desired.

Nutritional Data: Calories: 210 | Total Fat: 4.5g | Saturated Fat: 0.5g | Cholesterol: 0mg | Sodium: 80mg | Total Carbohydrates: 37g | Dietary Fiber: 5g | Sugars: 8g | Protein: 6g

Ginger-Pear Smoothie

Preparation Time: 10 minutes | Portion Size: 2 servings

Ingredients:
- 2 ripe pears, cored and roughly chopped
- 1-inch fresh ginger, peeled and minced
- 1 cup unsweetened almond milk (or any other non-dairy milk)
- 1 tbsp chia seeds
- 1 tbsp honey (or to taste, optional for added sweetness)
- A pinch of ground cinnamon
- 1/2 cup plain Greek yogurt or non-dairy yogurt alternative
- A handful of ice cubes (optional)

Instructions:

In a blender, combine the chopped pears, minced ginger, almond milk, chia seeds, honey (if using), and cinnamon. Blend on high until the mixture becomes smooth.

Add the Greek yogurt (or non-dairy alternative) and ice cubes if desired. Blend again until all ingredients are well combined and the smoothie reaches a creamy consistency. Pour the smoothie into glasses and serve immediately. You can sprinkle a dash of cinnamon on top for added garnish.

Nutritional Data: Calories: 165 | Total Fat: 2.5g | Saturated Fat: 0.3g | Cholesterol: 3mg | Sodium: 55mg | Total Carbohydrates: 32g | Dietary Fiber: 6g | Sugars: 20g | Protein: 6g

Avocado Toast on Sprouted Bread

Preparation Time: 5 minutes | Cooking Time: 2 minutes | Portion Size: 2 servings

Ingredients:
- 4 slices of sprouted grain bread
- 2 ripe avocados
- 1 tsp freshly squeezed lemon or lime juice
- A pinch of sea salt
- A pinch of black pepper
- Optional toppings: sliced radishes, sprouts, cherry tomatoes, or sliced cucumber

Instructions:
Start by toasting the sprouted grain bread slices to your preferred crispness.
While the bread is toasting, halve the avocados, remove the pits, and scoop the flesh into a bowl.
Mash the avocado flesh with a fork until smooth. You can leave some chunks if you prefer a more textured spread.
Mix in the freshly squeezed lemon or lime juice. Season with sea salt and black pepper.
Spread the mashed avocado mixture evenly over the toasted sprouted bread slices.
Top with your choice of optional toppings for additional texture and flavor.

Nutritional Data: Calories: 320 | Total Fat: 19g | Saturated Fat: 3g | Cholesterol: 0mg | Sodium: 150mg | Total Carbohydrates: 35g | Dietary Fiber: 13g | Sugars: 3g | Protein: 9g

Mint & Melon Medley

Preparation Time: 15 minutes | Portion Size: 4 servings

Ingredients:
- 2 cups honeydew melon, cubed
- 2 cups cantaloupe, cubed
- 2 cups watermelon, cubed
- 1/4 cup fresh mint leaves, finely chopped
- 1 tbsp freshly squeezed lemon juice
- 1 tbsp honey (optional, for added sweetness)
- A pinch of sea salt

Instructions:

In a large mixing bowl, combine the cubed honeydew, cantaloupe, and watermelon.

In a separate smaller bowl, whisk together the freshly squeezed lemon juice, honey (if using), and a pinch of sea salt.

Drizzle the lemon-honey mixture over the melon cubes and gently toss until well combined.

Sprinkle the finely chopped mint leaves over the melon mixture and give it one more gentle toss.

Chill in the refrigerator for about 10 minutes before serving. This step is optional but helps meld the flavors together and provides a refreshing chill to the dish.

Nutritional Data: Calories: 80 | Total Fat: 0.4g | Saturated Fat: 0.1g | Cholesterol: 0mg | Sodium: 30mg | Total Carbohydrates: 20g | Dietary Fiber: 1.5g | Sugars: 18g | Protein: 1.5g

Flaxseed Morning Muffins

Preparation Time: 20 minutes | Cooking Time: 25 minutes | Portion Size: 12 muffins

Ingredients:

- 2 cups whole wheat flour
- 1/2 cup ground flaxseeds
- 2 tsp baking powder
- 1/2 tsp baking soda
- 1/4 tsp sea salt
- 1/2 cup unsweetened applesauce
- 1/4 cup coconut oil, melted
- 1/2 cup honey or maple syrup
- 2 large eggs
- 1 tsp pure vanilla extract
- 1 cup unsweetened almond milk (or another non-dairy milk)
- 1/2 cup chopped nuts (such as walnuts or almonds), optional

Instructions:

Preheat your oven to 375°F (190°C). Line a muffin tin with paper liners or lightly grease.

In a large bowl, whisk together whole wheat flour, ground flaxseeds, baking powder, baking soda, and sea salt.

In a separate bowl, mix the applesauce, melted coconut oil, honey (or maple syrup), eggs, vanilla extract, and almond milk until well combined.

Pour the wet ingredients into the dry ingredient mixture and stir gently until just combined. If desired, fold in the chopped nuts.

Evenly divide the batter among the muffin cups.

Bake in the preheated oven for 20-25 minutes, or until a toothpick inserted into the center of a muffin comes out clean.

Allow the muffins to cool in the tin for about 5 minutes, then transfer to a wire rack to cool completely.

Nutritional Data: Calories: 190 | Total Fat: 7g | Saturated Fat: 3.5g | Cholesterol: 30mg | Sodium: 150mg | Total Carbohydrates: 28g | Dietary Fiber: 4g | Sugars: 12g | Protein: 5g

Quinoa Porridge

Preparation Time: 10 minutes | Cooking Time: 20 minutes | Portion Size: 4 servings

Ingredients:
- 1 cup quinoa, rinsed and drained
- 2 cups unsweetened almond milk (or another non-dairy milk)
- 1 cup water
- 1 tsp vanilla extract
- 1/4 tsp sea salt
- 2 tbsp chia seeds
- 1/4 cup raisins or dried cranberries (optional)
- 1/4 cup chopped nuts (such as almonds or walnuts)
- Fresh fruit (like berries or sliced bananas) for topping
- A drizzle of maple syrup or honey, for sweetness (optional)

Instructions:

In a medium-sized saucepan, combine quinoa, almond milk, water, vanilla extract, and sea salt. Bring the mixture to a boil over medium-high heat. Once boiling, reduce heat to low, cover, and let simmer for 15 minutes, or until the quinoa has absorbed most of the liquid and is tender. Remove from heat and stir in the chia seeds, raisins or dried cranberries (if using), and chopped nuts. Let the porridge sit for a few minutes to thicken, thanks to the chia seeds. Serve warm in bowls, topped with fresh fruit and a drizzle of maple syrup or honey if desired.

Nutritional Data: Calories: 260 | Total Fat: 7g | Saturated Fat: 0.5g | Cholesterol: 0mg | Sodium: 180mg | Total Carbohydrates: 40g | Dietary Fiber: 6g | Sugars: 10g | Protein: 8g

Banana & Almond Butter Oats

Preparation Time: 10 minutes (refrigeration time: 8 hours) | Portion Size: 2 servings

Ingredients:
- 1 cup rolled oats
- 1 ripe banana, mashed
- 1 tbsp chia seeds
- 2 tbsp almond butter
- 1 cup unsweetened almond milk (or another non-dairy milk)
- 1/2 tsp vanilla extract
- A pinch of sea salt
- Optional toppings: sliced bananas, a drizzle of honey, or a sprinkle of cinnamon

Instructions:

In a mixing bowl, combine the mashed banana, chia seeds, almond butter, almond milk, vanilla extract, and a pinch of salt. Stir until well mixed. Fold in the rolled oats, ensuring they are fully submerged in the liquid. Divide the mixture between two jars or airtight containers, sealing them tightly. Refrigerate the oats overnight, or for at least 8 hours. In the morning, give the oats a good stir. If the mixture is too thick, add a splash more almond milk until you reach your desired consistency. Top with additional banana slices, a drizzle of honey, or a sprinkle of cinnamon if desired. Enjoy cold, or heat in the microwave for a warm breakfast treat.

Nutritional Data: Calories: 360 | Total Fat: 10g | Saturated Fat: 1g | Cholesterol: 0mg | Sodium: 150mg | Total Carbohydrates: 58g | Dietary Fiber: 9g | Sugars: 10g | Protein: 10g

Coconut & Blueberry Chia Pudding

Preparation Time: 15 minutes   (refrigeration time: 4 hours) | Portion Size: 3 servings

Ingredients:
- 1/4 cup chia seeds
- 1 cup unsweetened coconut milk (from a carton)
- 1/2 cup full-fat canned coconut milk
- 1 tbsp maple syrup (adjust to taste)
- 1 tsp vanilla extract
- 1 cup fresh blueberries
- Optional toppings: shredded coconut, additional blueberries, or a sprinkle of cinnamon

Instructions:

In a mixing bowl, combine the chia seeds, unsweetened coconut milk, full-fat canned coconut milk, maple syrup, and vanilla extract. Whisk until well combined.

Allow the mixture to sit for about 10 minutes, then stir again to ensure even distribution of the chia seeds.

Fold in the fresh blueberries.

Divide the mixture between three jars or airtight containers, sealing them tightly.

Refrigerate for at least 4 hours, or until the pudding has set.

Before serving, give the pudding a good stir to break up any clumps of chia seeds.

Top with shredded coconut, additional blueberries, or a sprinkle of cinnamon if desired.

Nutritional Data: Calories: 250 | Total Fat: 15g | Saturated Fat: 10g | Cholesterol: 0mg | Sodium: 30mg | Total Carbohydrates: 24g | Dietary Fiber: 7g | Sugars: 12g | Protein: 4g

Greens Morning Juice

Preparation Time: 10 minutes   (No cooking required) | Portion Size: 2 servings

Ingredients:
- 1 large cucumber, peeled and chopped
- 2 handfuls of baby spinach
- 1 green apple, cored and sliced (leave the peel on)
- 1/2 fennel bulb, chopped
- 1 inch piece of fresh ginger, peeled
- 1/2 lemon, peeled
- 1 cup of coconut water or filtered water

Instructions:

Wash and prepare all the ingredients as indicated above. Start your juicer and feed the cucumber, spinach, green apple, fennel, ginger, and lemon through it one by one. After juicing, pour the juice into a blender and add the coconut water or filtered water. Blend for about 10-15 seconds to combine everything well.
Pour into glasses and drink immediately to get the most nutritional benefits.

Nutritional Data: Calories: 90 | Total Fat: 0.5g | Saturated Fat: 0g | Cholesterol: 0mg | Sodium: 65mg | Total Carbohydrates: 21g | Dietary Fiber: 4g | Sugars: 13g | Protein: 2g

Cucumber and Zucchini Smoothie

Preparation Time: 5 minutes | Cooking Time: 0 minutes | Portion Size: 2 servings

Ingredients:
- 1 medium cucumber, peeled and chopped
- 1 small zucchini, chopped
- 1/2 cup unsweetened almond milk (or other non-dairy milk)
- 1 tbsp chia seeds
- 1 tbsp fresh mint leaves (optional)
- 1 tbsp honey or maple syrup (optional, for sweetness)
- A handful of ice cubes

Instructions:

In a blender, combine the cucumber, zucchini, almond milk, chia seeds, mint leaves (if using), and honey or maple syrup (if desired). Blend until smooth and creamy, adding ice cubes for a cooler, thicker consistency.
Pour into glasses and serve immediately.

Nutritional Data:
Calories: 90 | Total Fat: 3g | Saturated Fat: 0g | Cholesterol: 0mg | Sodium: 60mg | Total Carbohydrates: 15g | Dietary Fiber: 4g | Sugars: 5g | Protein: 3g

Cinnamon Rice Cereal Delight

Preparation Time: 5 minutes | Cooking Time: 10 minutes | Portion Size: 2 servings

Ingredients:

- 1 cup of rice cereal
- 1 1/2 cups of unsweetened almond milk
- 1/2 teaspoon of ground cinnamon
- 1 tablespoon of honey (optional)
- 1/2 cup of sliced bananas
- 1/4 cup of chopped almonds

Instructions:

In a saucepan, combine the rice cereal and almond milk. Cook over medium heat, stirring constantly, until the mixture thickens, about 5-7 minutes. Remove from heat and stir in the ground cinnamon. Add honey if desired for sweetness. Divide the cereal mixture into two serving bowls. Top with sliced bananas and chopped almonds.

Nutritional Data:

Calories: 250 | Fat: 8g | Carbohydrates: 42g | Fiber: 5g | Sugar: 12g | Protein: 5g

Note: Nutritional values are approximate and may vary based on specific ingredients used.

Oatmeal with Apple and Chia Seeds

Preparation Time: 5 minutes | Cooking Time: 10 minutes | Portion Size: 2 servings

Ingredients:

- 1 cup rolled oats
- 2 cups unsweetened almond milk (or other non-dairy milk)
- 1 medium apple, peeled and diced
- 1 tbsp chia seeds
- 1/2 tsp ground cinnamon
- 1 tbsp maple syrup (optional)
- A pinch of salt
- Fresh apple slices or chopped nuts for garnish (optional)

Instructions:

In a medium saucepan, bring the almond milk to a simmer over medium heat. Stir in the rolled oats and diced apple. Cook for about 5-7 minutes, stirring occasionally, until the oats are soft and the mixture thickens. Stir in the chia seeds, ground cinnamon, maple syrup (if using), and a pinch of salt. Cook for an additional 2-3 minutes until the chia seeds have absorbed some liquid and the oatmeal is creamy.

Remove from heat and serve warm, garnished with fresh apple slices or chopped nuts if desired.

Nutritional Data:

Calories: 230 | Total Fat: 6g | Saturated Fat: 1g | Cholesterol: 0mg | Sodium: 100mg | Total Carbohydrates: 40g | Dietary Fiber: 8g | Sugars: 10g | Protein: 6g

Blueberry and Almond Milk Smoothie

Preparation Time: 5 minutes | Cooking Time: 0 minutes | Portion Size: 2 servings

Ingredients:
- 1 cup fresh or frozen blueberries
- 1 cup unsweetened almond milk
- 1 tbsp chia seeds
- 1/2 tsp vanilla extract
- 1 tbsp honey or maple syrup (optional)
- A handful of ice cubes (optional)

Instructions:

In a blender, combine the blueberries, almond milk, chia seeds, vanilla extract, and honey or maple syrup (if using). Blend on high until smooth and creamy. Add ice cubes for a colder, thicker smoothie if desired.

Nutritional Data:

Calories: 120 | Total Fat: 4g | Saturated Fat: 0g | Cholesterol: 0mg | Sodium: 90mg | Total Carbohydrates: 21g | Dietary Fiber: 5g | Sugars: 10g | Protein: 3g

Buckwheat & Berry Bliss Bowl

Preparation Time: 10 minutes | Cooking Time: 20 minutes (if buckwheat is uncooked) | Portion Size: 2 servings

Ingredients:
- 1 cup cooked buckwheat groats
- 1/2 cup fresh blueberries
- 1/2 cup fresh strawberries, sliced
- 1 tablespoon chia seeds
- 2 tablespoons unsweetened almond milk or any non-dairy milk
- 1 tablespoon honey or maple syrup (optional)
- A sprinkle of unsweetened coconut flakes
- A pinch of ground cinnamon

Instructions:

If you're starting with uncooked buckwheat, rinse the groats thoroughly under cool water. In a saucepan, bring 2 cups of water to a boil, add the buckwheat, reduce the heat, and simmer for about 20 minutes or until the buckwheat is tender and the water is absorbed. Let it cool. In a bowl, combine the cooled buckwheat groats with almond milk to give it a slightly creamy texture. Gently fold in the blueberries and sliced strawberries. Drizzle with honey or maple syrup for a touch of sweetness if desired. Top with chia seeds, a sprinkle of coconut flakes, and a pinch of ground cinnamon. Stir gently to combine and serve immediately.

Nutritional Data: Calories: 265 | Total Fat: 3g | Saturated Fat: 0.5g | Cholesterol: 0mg | Sodium: 15mg | Total Carbohydrates: 54g | Dietary Fiber: 8g | Sugars: 12g | Protein: 8g

Refined-Sugar-Free Apple & Cinnamon Crepes

Preparation Time: 15 minutes | Cooking Time: 20 minutes | Portion Size: 4 servings (2 crepes per serving)

Ingredients:

For the crepes:

- 1 cup whole wheat flour or spelt flour
- 1 1/2 cups unsweetened almond milk (or another non-dairy milk)
- 2 large eggs
- 1 tablespoon melted coconut oil or unsalted butter, plus more for frying
- A pinch of salt

For the filling:

- 2 large apples, peeled, cored, and thinly sliced
- 1 teaspoon ground cinnamon
- 1 tablespoon honey or maple syrup
- 1/2 teaspoon pure vanilla extract
- Coconut oil or unsalted butter for sautéing

Instructions:

Prepare the Crepe Batter: In a mixing bowl, whisk together the flour, almond milk, eggs, melted coconut oil, and salt until smooth. Allow the batter to rest for about 10 minutes.

Cook the Apples: In a skillet over medium heat, melt a small amount of coconut oil or butter. Add the sliced apples, cinnamon, and honey. Cook, stirring occasionally, until the apples are softened and slightly caramelized, about 7-8 minutes. Stir in the vanilla extract. Remove from heat and set aside.

Cook the Crepes: Heat a non-stick skillet or crepe pan over medium heat. Add a little coconut oil or butter to coat the pan lightly. Pour in a quarter cup of the crepe batter and tilt the pan, spreading the batter thinly across the bottom. Cook until the edges of the crepe lift easily and the bottom is lightly golden, about 2 minutes. Flip and cook for another 1-2 minutes on the other side. Transfer to a plate and repeat with the remaining batter.

Assemble the Crepes: Lay a crepe flat on a plate. Spoon some of the apple filling down the center. Fold the sides over the filling. Repeat with the remaining crepes and filling.

Serve: Serve the crepes warm, with a drizzle of honey or maple syrup if desired.

Nutritional Data: Calories: 225 | Total Fat: 6g | Saturated Fat: 3g | Cholesterol: 93mg | Sodium: 75mg | Total Carbohydrates: 37g | Dietary Fiber: 6g | Sugars: 12g | Protein: 7g

Tofu & Spinach Breakfast Scramble

Preparation Time: 10 minutes | Cooking Time: 15 minutes | Portion Size: 4 servings

Ingredients:

- 1 block (14 oz.) firm tofu, pressed and crumbled
- 2 tbsp olive oil
- 1 small onion, finely chopped
- 2 cloves garlic, minced
- 2 cups fresh spinach, washed and chopped
- 1/4 tsp turmeric powder (for color and added health benefits)
- 1/2 tsp black salt (kala namak) or regular salt (black salt gives an eggy flavor)
- Freshly ground black pepper to taste
- Optional: 1/4 cup nutritional yeast (for a cheesy flavor)

Instructions:

Begin by pressing the tofu to remove excess water. Use a tofu press or place it between two clean kitchen towels and set a heavy pan on top. Let it sit for about 10 minutes. While the tofu is pressing, heat olive oil in a large skillet over medium heat. Add the chopped onion and sauté until translucent. Add the minced garlic and sauté for another minute until fragrant. Crumble the pressed tofu into the skillet. Use a fork or your hands to break it into small, scrambled egg-sized pieces. Sprinkle the turmeric over the tofu and stir well to combine, giving the tofu a yellowish hue. Add the chopped spinach and cook until the spinach has wilted. Season with black salt or regular salt, black pepper, and nutritional yeast if using. Stir well to ensure all ingredients are well combined. Cook for another 5-7 minutes, stirring occasionally until the tofu is heated through and has taken on the flavors of the seasonings. Taste and adjust seasonings if necessary. Serve hot with whole grain toast or as a filling for a breakfast wrap.

Nutritional Data (per serving): Calories: 180 | Total Fat: 12g | Saturated Fat: 2g | Cholesterol: 0mg | Sodium: 300mg | Total Carbohydrates: 7g | Dietary Fiber: 3g | Sugars: 2g | Protein: 13g |

Whole Grain Toast with Pumpkin Cream and Flax Seeds

Preparation Time: 10 minutes | Cooking Time: 5 minutes | Portion Size: 2 servings

Ingredients:

- 2 slices whole grain bread
- 1/2 cup cooked pumpkin purée (unsweetened)
- 1 tbsp flax seeds
- 1 tbsp olive oil
- 1/4 tsp ground cinnamon
- 1 tsp honey or maple syrup (optional)
- A pinch of salt
- Fresh parsley for garnish (optional)

Instructions:

Toast the slices of whole grain bread to your preferred crispness. In a small bowl, mix together the pumpkin purée, olive oil, ground cinnamon, honey or maple syrup (if using), and a pinch of salt. Spread the pumpkin cream evenly over the toasted bread slices. Sprinkle with flax seeds and garnish with fresh parsley if desired.

Nutritional Data:

Calories: 180 | Total Fat: 9g | Saturated Fat: 1g | Cholesterol: 0mg | Sodium: 180mg | Total Carbohydrates: 22g | Dietary Fiber: 5g | Sugars: 4g | Protein: 4g

Whole Wheat Couscous with Chickpeas and Roasted Vegetables

Preparation Time: 15 minutes | Cooking Time: 25 minutes | Portion Size: 4 servings

Ingredients:

- 1 cup whole wheat couscous
- 1 1/4 cups low-sodium vegetable broth
- 1 medium zucchini, diced
- 1 red bell pepper, diced (optional for those who tolerate it)
- 1 medium carrot, peeled and diced
- 1 small eggplant, diced
- 1 (15 oz) can chickpeas, drained and rinsed
- 2 tbsp olive oil
- 1 tsp dried thyme
- 1 tsp dried oregano
- Salt and pepper, to taste
- Fresh parsley, chopped (optional, for garnish)

Instructions:

Preheat the oven to 400°F (200°C). In a large bowl, toss the zucchini, red bell pepper (if using), carrot, and eggplant with olive oil, thyme, oregano, salt, and pepper. Spread the vegetables on a baking sheet and roast in the oven for 20-25 minutes, stirring halfway, until tender and slightly caramelized. While the vegetables are roasting, bring the vegetable broth to a boil in a medium saucepan. Remove from heat, stir in the couscous, cover, and let it sit for 5 minutes. Fluff with a fork. Once the vegetables are ready, mix the roasted vegetables and chickpeas into the couscous. Garnish with fresh parsley if desired and serve warm.

Nutritional Data:

Calories: 280 | Total Fat: 8g | Saturated Fat: 1g | Cholesterol: 0mg | Sodium: 250mg | Total Carbohydrates: 44g | Dietary Fiber: 9g | Sugars: 6g | Protein: 9g

Omega-Rich Chia & Hemp Seed Parfait

Preparation Time: 10 minutes (no cooking required) | Portion Size: 2 servings

Ingredients:

- 1/4 cup chia seeds
- 1 cup almond milk (or any non-dairy milk of choice)
- 2 tablespoons hemp seeds
- 1 tablespoon honey or maple syrup (optional)
- 1/2 teaspoon vanilla extract
- 1/2 cup fresh blueberries
- 1/2 cup fresh strawberries, sliced
- 2 tablespoons unsweetened shredded coconut

Instructions:

In a mixing bowl, combine chia seeds and almond milk. Stir well and let it sit for at least 30 minutes to an hour (or overnight in the refrigerator) until it thickens to a pudding-like consistency.

Once the chia pudding is ready, stir in hemp seeds, sweetener (if using), and vanilla extract.

In serving glasses or bowls, layer a portion of the chia and hemp seed mixture, followed by a layer of blueberries, and then strawberries.

Repeat the layers until all ingredients are used up, finishing with a sprinkle of shredded coconut on top.

Serve immediately or refrigerate for later. Enjoy this nutrient-dense, omega-rich parfait!

Tip: If you prefer a smoother texture, you can blend the chia seed and almond milk mixture until smooth before layering with fruits.

Nutritional Data (per serving): Calories: 280 | Total Fat: 17g | Saturated Fat: 3.5g | Cholesterol: 0mg | Sodium: 90mg | Total Carbohydrates: 25g | Dietary Fiber: 12g | Sugars: 10g | Protein: 8g | Omega-3 fatty acids: 2.5g | Omega-6 fatty acids: 2g.

As we wrap up our exploration of breakfast recipes, our wish is for you to embark on each day with a sense of enthusiasm, fueled by meals that nurture both body and soul. Gone are the days when breakfast felt like a gamble, each bite potentially paving the way for unease. With these carefully curated dishes, mornings are transformed into moments of serenity and satisfaction. May every sunrise be greeted with anticipation, every breakfast plate be a canvas of culinary art, and every day commence with confidence and comfort. Onward to a day brimming with potential and free from digestive dismay!

Chapter 5: Lunch

Lunch holds a special place in our daily routine, serving as a pivotal moment that bridges the gap between the morning's endeavors and the afternoon's undertakings. It's an opportunity to pause, recharge, refocus, and revitalize our minds and bodies. However, for those who grapple with the challenges of acid reflux, this midday meal can sometimes feel like a delicate balancing act, where the need for nourishment must be carefully weighed against the fear of triggering discomfort.

In this enlightening "Lunch Recipes" chapter, we've embarked on a culinary journey to create dishes that not only tantalize the taste buds but also respect and support your digestive well-being. Here, flavor seamlessly marries function, offering you a medley of meals that satiate your hunger while ensuring a harmonious and gentle digestive journey for the hours to come.

These recipes have been thoughtfully curated to reduce the risk of acid reflux-related discomfort while embracing the pleasure of food. They demonstrate that lunch can be both a satisfying and supportive experience, one where each bite not only delights your palate but also nourishes your body without fear of digestive distress. So, as you explore this chapter, envision lunch as more than just a meal—it's an opportunity to care for your well-being while savoring the flavors of life.

Recipes

Brown Rice Bowl with Grilled Vegetables

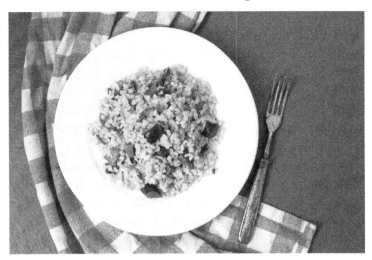

Preparation Time: 10 minutes | Cooking Time: 30 minutes | Portion Size: 4 servings

Ingredients:

- 1 cup brown rice, rinsed
- 2 cups water
- 1 medium zucchini, sliced
- 1 red bell pepper, sliced (optional for those who tolerate it)
- 1 large carrot, peeled and sliced
- 1 small eggplant, sliced
- 2 tbsp olive oil
- 1 tsp dried oregano
- 1 tsp dried thyme
- Salt and pepper, to taste

Instructions:

In a medium saucepan, combine the brown rice and water. Bring to a boil, then reduce heat, cover, and simmer for about 25-30 minutes or until the rice is tender and water is absorbed. Remove from heat and let it sit for 5 minutes before fluffing with a fork. While the rice is cooking, preheat your grill (or grill pan) over medium heat. In a bowl, toss the zucchini, bell pepper (if using), carrot, and eggplant with olive oil, oregano, thyme, salt, and pepper. Grill the vegetables for about 3-4 minutes on each side or until they are tender and have nice grill marks. Divide the cooked brown rice into bowls and top with the grilled vegetables.

Nutritional Data:
Calories: 220 | Total Fat: 8g | Saturated Fat: 1g | Cholesterol: 0mg | Sodium: 25mg | Total Carbohydrates: 35g | Dietary Fiber: 5g | Sugars: 5g | Protein: 5g

Spinach, Quinoa, and Avocado Salad

Preparation Time: 10 minutes | Cooking Time: 15 minutes | Portion Size: 4 servings

Ingredients:

- 1 cup quinoa, rinsed
- 2 cups water
- 4 cups fresh baby spinach
- 1 large avocado, diced
- 1 small cucumber, diced
- 1 tbsp olive oil
- 1 tbsp lemon juice (optional for those who tolerate it)
- Salt and pepper, to taste

Instructions:

In a medium saucepan, bring the quinoa and water to a boil. Reduce the heat to low, cover, and let it simmer for about 12-15 minutes, or until the quinoa is cooked and the water is absorbed. Fluff with a fork and set aside to cool. In a large bowl, combine the spinach, diced avocado, and cucumber. Add the cooked quinoa to the salad and toss gently. Drizzle with olive oil and, if tolerated, lemon juice. Season with salt and pepper to taste.

Nutritional Data:
Calories: 250 | Total Fat: 12g | Saturated Fat: 1.5g | Cholesterol: 0mg | Sodium: 20mg | Total Carbohydrates: 30g | Dietary Fiber: 7g | Sugars: 3g | Protein: 7g

Cannellini Bean and Carrot Soup

Preparation Time: 10 minutes | Cooking Time: 25 minutes | Portion Size: 4 servings

Ingredients:

- 1 tbsp olive oil
- 1 medium onion, finely chopped (optional, or use leek for a milder option)
- 2 garlic cloves, minced (optional for those who tolerate it)
- 4 large carrots, peeled and sliced
- 1 (15 oz) can cannellini beans, drained and rinsed
- 4 cups low-sodium vegetable broth
- 1 tsp dried thyme
- Salt and pepper, to taste
- Fresh parsley, for garnish (optional)

Instructions:

In a large pot, heat the olive oil over medium heat. If using onion and garlic, sauté them until soft and translucent, about 5 minutes. Add the sliced carrots and cook for another 3 minutes, stirring occasionally.

Add the cannellini beans, vegetable broth, thyme, salt, and pepper. Bring to a boil, then reduce heat and simmer for 20 minutes, or until the carrots are tender. Use an immersion blender to puree the soup to your desired consistency, or transfer to a blender in batches for a smoother texture.

Adjust seasoning with salt and pepper, if necessary. Garnish with fresh parsley and serve warm.

Nutritional Data:

Calories: 180 | Total Fat: 4g | Saturated Fat: 0.5g | Cholesterol: 0mg | Sodium: 290mg | Total Carbohydrates: 30g | Dietary Fiber: 8g | Sugars: 6g | Protein: 7g

Tender Turmeric Chicken Wraps

Preparation Time: 20 minutes | Cooking Time: 15 minutes | Portion Size: 4 servings

---

Ingredients:

- 1 pound (450g) boneless, skinless chicken breast, thinly sliced
- 1 tablespoon ground turmeric
- 2 tablespoons olive oil
- 4 whole grain tortilla wraps
- 1 avocado, sliced
- 1 cucumber, sliced thinly
- 1/2 cup Greek yogurt (or a dairy-free alternative)
- Salt and pepper to taste
- Fresh cilantro for garnish (optional)
- Fresh lime wedges for serving (optional)

Instructions:

Marinate the Chicken: In a bowl, combine the chicken slices with turmeric, salt, and pepper. Ensure the chicken is well-coated and allow it to marinate for at least 15 minutes.

Cook the Chicken: In a skillet over medium-high heat, warm the olive oil. Add the marinated chicken and cook until it is thoroughly cooked and slightly golden on each side, approximately 5-7 minutes.

Prepare the Wraps: While the chicken is cooking, lay out the whole-grain wraps and spread a generous dollop of Greek yogurt (or alternative) on each.

Add Veggies: Layer avocado slices and cucumber slices evenly among the wraps.

Add the Chicken: Once cooked, distribute the chicken slices among the wraps.

Fold and Serve: Carefully fold the wraps and serve with a sprinkle of fresh cilantro and a squeeze of lime, if desired.

Nutritional Data: Calories: 400 | Total Fat: 18g | Saturated Fat: 3g | Cholesterol: 85mg | Sodium: 230mg | Total Carbohydrates: 26g | Dietary Fiber: 6g | Sugars: 3g | Protein: 35g

Zucchini Noodles with Pesto

Preparation Time: 15 minutes | Cooking Time: 5 minutes | Portion Size: 4 servings

Ingredients:

- 4 medium zucchinis, spiralized into noodles
- 1 cup fresh basil leaves
- 1/2 cup spinach leaves
- 1/3 cup walnuts (or pine nuts)
- 1/3 cup grated Parmesan cheese (or nutritional yeast for a dairy-free alternative)
- 1/4 cup extra virgin olive oil
- 2 cloves garlic
- Salt and freshly ground black pepper to taste
- Cherry tomatoes, halved, for garnish (optional)

Instructions:

Prepare the Pesto: In a food processor, combine basil, spinach, walnuts, garlic, and Parmesan cheese. Blend until smooth. Gradually add olive oil while the processor is running, until you get a creamy consistency. Season with salt and pepper.

Prepare the Zucchini Noodles: Using a spiralizer or a julienne peeler, turn the zucchinis into noodles. If you don't have a spiralizer, you can use a regular vegetable peeler to create wide zucchini ribbons.

Sauté the Zucchini Noodles: Heat a large skillet over medium heat. Add the zucchini noodles and sauté for about 2-3 minutes, just until the noodles are tender. Be careful not to overcook, as they can become too soft.

Combine Pesto and Zucchini Noodles: Remove the skillet from the heat. Add the pesto to the zucchini noodles and toss well to combine.

Serve: Divide the zucchini noodles among plates. Garnish with cherry tomatoes if desired.

Nutritional Data: Calories: 250 | Total Fat: 20g | Saturated Fat: 3g | Cholesterol: 7mg | Sodium: 150mg | Total Carbohydrates: 12g | Dietary Fiber: 4g | Sugars: 6g | Protein: 8g

Spinach & Tofu Curry

Preparation Time: 20 minutes | Cooking Time: 25 minutes | Portion Size: 4 servings

Ingredients:

- 1 block (14 oz) firm tofu, drained, pressed, and cubed
- 4 cups fresh spinach leaves, washed and roughly chopped
- 1 can (13.5 oz) light coconut milk
- 2 tbsp olive oil
- 1 large onion, finely chopped
- 2 cloves garlic, minced
- 1-inch ginger, grated
- 1 tsp ground turmeric
- 1/2 tsp ground cumin
- 1/2 tsp ground coriander
- Salt to taste
- Fresh cilantro, chopped (for garnish)

Instructions:

Sauté the Tofu: In a large skillet, heat 1 tablespoon of olive oil over medium heat. Add the tofu cubes and sauté until they are golden brown on all sides. Remove the tofu and set it aside. Prepare the Curry Base: In the same skillet, add the remaining olive oil and sauté onions until they're translucent. Add the minced garlic and grated ginger and cook for an additional 2 minutes. Spices and Coconut Milk: Sprinkle the turmeric, cumin, and coriander into the skillet. Stir well, ensuring the onions are well coated. Pour in the coconut milk, stirring to combine. Add Spinach and Tofu: Once the coconut milk starts to simmer, fold in the chopped spinach. Allow the spinach to wilt, which should take about 3-5 minutes. Gently add the sautéed tofu cubes to the skillet and let everything simmer for an additional 10 minutes, allowing the flavors to meld. Season and Serve: Season the curry with salt to taste. Once done, serve the curry in bowls, garnishing with fresh chopped cilantro.

Nutritional Data: Calories: 280 | Total Fat: 20g | Saturated Fat: 9g | Cholesterol: 0mg | Sodium: 80mg | Total Carbohydrates: 10g | Dietary Fiber: 3g | Sugars: 3g | Protein: 17g

Rustic Root Vegetable Medley

Preparation Time: 15 minutes | Cooking Time: 45 minutes | Portion Size: 4 servings

Ingredients:

- 2 medium carrots, peeled and diced
- 2 medium parsnips, peeled and diced
- 1 large sweet potato, peeled and diced
- 1 medium turnip, peeled and diced
- 2 tbsp olive oil
- 2 tsp fresh rosemary, finely chopped
- Salt to taste
- Freshly ground black pepper to taste
- Fresh parsley, chopped (for garnish)

Instructions:

Preheat the Oven: Preheat your oven to 400°F (200°C).

Prepare the Vegetables: In a large mixing bowl, combine the diced carrots, parsnips, sweet potato, and turnip.

Season: Drizzle the vegetables with olive oil, then sprinkle with chopped rosemary, salt, and black pepper. Toss well to ensure all the vegetables are well coated.

Roast: Spread the seasoned vegetables evenly on a baking tray lined with parchment paper. Place the tray in the preheated oven and roast for 40-45 minutes or until the vegetables are tender and have a light golden color. Turn the vegetables halfway through to ensure even cooking.

Serve: Once cooked, remove the vegetables from the oven and transfer them to a serving dish. Garnish with fresh chopped parsley before serving.

Nutritional Data: Calories: 200 | Total Fat: 7g | Saturated Fat: 1g | Cholesterol: 0mg | Sodium: 80mg | Total Carbohydrates: 33g | Dietary Fiber: 7g | Sugars: 8g | Protein: 2g

Steamed Sea Bass Fillet with Fennel

Preparation Time: 10 minutes | Cooking Time: 15 minutes | Portion Size: 4 servings

Ingredients:

- 4 sea bass fillets (about 150g each)
- 1 large fennel bulb, thinly sliced
- 1 tbsp olive oil
- 1 tsp dried thyme
- Salt and pepper, to taste
- 1 lemon, sliced (optional, for those who tolerate it)

Instructions:

Prepare a steamer by bringing water to a boil in a pot or steamer. In a bowl, toss the sliced fennel with olive oil, thyme, salt, and pepper. Place the sea bass fillets and fennel slices in the steamer. Steam for about 10-12 minutes, or until the fish is opaque and flakes easily with a fork. Optionally, serve with lemon slices on the side for those who can tolerate citrus.

Nutritional Data:

Calories: 240 | Total Fat: 10g | Saturated Fat: 2g | Cholesterol: 60mg | Sodium: 80mg | Total Carbohydrates: 6g | Dietary Fiber: 2g | Sugars: 2g | Protein: 30g

Rice Pilaf with Almonds

Preparation Time: 10 minutes | Cooking Time: 25 minutes | Portion Size: 4 servings

Ingredients:

- 1 cup long-grain white rice
- 2 1/4 cups low-sodium vegetable broth
- 1/2 cup almonds, slivered and toasted
- 1 small onion, finely chopped
- 2 tbsp extra-virgin olive oil
- 1 bay leaf
- Salt to taste
- 1 tbsp fresh parsley, chopped (for garnish)

Instructions:

Saute the Onions: In a medium saucepan, heat the olive oil over medium heat. Add the chopped onions and sauté until translucent and soft, about 5 minutes. Toast the Rice: Add the rice to the saucepan and stir well, ensuring each grain is coated with the oil. Toast the rice for about 2 minutes until it starts giving off a nutty aroma. Add Broth & Seasonings: Pour in the vegetable broth and add the bay leaf. Season with a pinch of salt, then stir to combine. Cook the Rice: Bring the mixture to a boil. Once boiling, reduce the heat to low, cover the saucepan with a lid, and let it simmer for approximately 20 minutes, or until the rice is cooked and the liquid is absorbed.

Add Almonds & Serve: Once the rice is done, remove it from heat and discard the bay leaf. Fluff the rice with a fork and fold in the toasted almond slivers. Transfer the rice pilaf to a serving dish, garnish with fresh parsley, and serve.

Nutritional Data: Calories: 280 | Total Fat: 12g | Saturated Fat: 1.5g | Cholesterol: 0mg | Sodium: 150mg | Total Carbohydrates: 37g | Dietary Fiber: 2g | Sugars: 2g | Protein: 6g

Hummus & Pita

Preparation Time: 10 minutes   (unless toasting pita) | Portion Size: 6 servings

Ingredients:
- 1 can (15 oz) chickpeas (garbanzo beans), drained and rinsed
- 3 tbsp tahini (sesame paste)
- 2 tbsp extra-virgin olive oil
- 1 clove garlic, minced
- Juice of 1 lemon
- Salt to taste
- 1/4 cup water (or more for desired consistency)
- 1/4 tsp ground cumin (optional for flavor)
- 6 whole grain pita bread rounds
- Olive oil (for toasting, optional)
- Fresh parsley, finely chopped for garnish

Instructions:

Blend the Ingredients: In a food processor, combine chickpeas, tahini, olive oil, minced garlic, lemon juice, salt, and ground cumin (if using). Blend until smooth.

Adjust Consistency: While the food processor is running, slowly add water until you achieve your desired consistency.

Toast the Pita (Optional): If you prefer toasted pita, brush the pita bread rounds lightly with olive oil. Place them in a preheated oven at 375°F (190°C) or on a grill for about 2-3 minutes each side until they are slightly crispy.

Serve: Transfer the hummus to a serving bowl, create a small well in the center, and drizzle a bit of olive oil in the well. Garnish with fresh parsley. Serve with pita bread on the side.

Nutritional Data: Calories: 250 | Total Fat: 8g | Saturated Fat: 1g | Cholesterol: 0mg | Sodium: 300mg | Total Carbohydrates: 36g | Dietary Fiber: 6g | Sugars: 1g | Protein: 9g

Baked Quinoa and Spinach Patties

Preparation Time: 15 minutes | Cooking Time: 25 minutes | Portion Size: 4 servings

Ingredients:
- 1 cup cooked quinoa
- 2 cups fresh spinach, chopped
- 1/2 cup breadcrumbs (whole wheat or gluten-free)
- 1/4 cup grated Parmesan cheese (optional)

- 1 egg, lightly beaten
- 1 tbsp olive oil
- 1 tsp dried oregano
- 1 tsp dried basil
- Salt and pepper, to taste

Instructions:

Preheat the oven to 375°F (190°C) and line a baking sheet with parchment paper. In a large bowl, combine the cooked quinoa, chopped spinach, breadcrumbs, Parmesan (if using), beaten egg, olive oil, oregano, basil, salt, and pepper. Mix well until all ingredients are evenly combined. Form the mixture into small patties, about the size of your palm, and place them on the prepared baking sheet. Bake in the preheated oven for 20-25 minutes, flipping halfway through, until the patties are golden brown and firm.

Nutritional Data:

Calories: 220 | Total Fat: 9g | Saturated Fat: 2g | Cholesterol: 60mg | Sodium: 150mg | Total Carbohydrates: 24g | Dietary Fiber: 4g | Sugars: 2g | Protein: 10g

Broccoli & Quinoa Bowl

Preparation Time: 10 minutes | Cooking Time: 20 minutes | Portion Size: 4 servings

Ingredients:
- 1 cup quinoa, rinsed and drained
- 2 cups water or low-sodium vegetable broth
- 2 tbsp extra-virgin olive oil
- 2 cups broccoli florets
- 2 cloves garlic, minced
- Salt to taste
- 1/4 cup almonds, chopped
- 2 green onions, sliced
- Lemon zest from 1 lemon
- Fresh parsley, chopped for garnish

Instructions:

Cook the Quinoa: In a medium-sized pot, bring the water or vegetable broth to a boil. Add the quinoa, reduce the heat to low, cover, and simmer for about 15 minutes or until the quinoa is cooked and the liquid is absorbed. Fluff with a fork and set aside.

Prepare the Broccoli: In a large skillet, heat the olive oil over medium heat. Add the minced garlic and sauté until fragrant. Add the broccoli florets and cook until they are bright green and slightly tender, about 5-7 minutes.

Mix and Serve: Add the cooked quinoa to the skillet and mix well with the broccoli. Season with salt to taste. Transfer to serving bowls and top with chopped almonds, green onions, lemon zest, and a garnish of fresh parsley.

Nutritional Data: Calories: 275 | Total Fat: 10g | Saturated Fat: 1.5g | Cholesterol: 0mg | Sodium: 55mg | Total Carbohydrates: 38g | Dietary Fiber: 6g | Sugars: 2g | Protein: 10g

Butternut Squash Soup

Preparation Time: 15 minutes | Cooking Time: 30 minutes | Portion Size: 4 servings

Ingredients:

- 1 medium butternut squash, peeled and diced
- 1 tablespoon olive oil
- 1 small onion, chopped
- 2 cloves garlic, minced
- 1 tablespoon fresh ginger, grated
- 4 cups low-sodium vegetable broth
- 1/2 teaspoon ground turmeric
- Salt and black pepper to taste
- 1 can (14 oz) coconut milk
- Fresh cilantro, for garnish
- Pumpkin seeds, for garnish

Instructions:

Roast the Squash: Preheat your oven to 400°F (200°C). Place the diced butternut squash on a baking sheet, lightly coat with olive oil, and roast for about 20 minutes until it's soft and slightly caramelized.

Prepare the Base: In a large pot, heat the olive oil over medium heat. Add the chopped onion and sauté until translucent. Add the minced garlic and grated ginger, and sauté for an additional 1-2 minutes until fragrant.

Add the Squash: Incorporate the roasted butternut squash to the pot and stir well to combine with the onion, garlic, and ginger.

Add the Liquids: Pour in the vegetable broth and bring the mixture to a boil. Lower the heat and let it simmer for about 10 minutes. Add the turmeric, salt, and black pepper, and stir well.

Blend the Soup: Using an immersion blender, blend the soup until it's smooth and creamy. Alternatively, you can transfer the soup to a blender, blend in batches, and return it to the pot.

Add Coconut Milk: Stir in the coconut milk and simmer for an additional 5 minutes. Adjust seasoning as needed.

Serve: Ladle the soup into bowls and garnish with fresh cilantro and pumpkin seeds before serving.

Nutritional Data: Calories: 220 | Total Fat: 12g | Saturated Fat: 8g | Cholesterol: 0mg | Sodium: 180mg | Total Carbohydrates: 29g | Dietary Fiber: 5g | Sugars: 7g | Protein: 3g

Polenta with Sautéed Greens

Preparation Time: 10 minutes | Cooking Time: 25 minutes | Portion Size: 4 servings

Ingredients:

- 1 cup polenta (corn grits)
- 4 cups low-sodium vegetable broth or water
- 1 tablespoon olive oil
- 4 cups mixed greens (spinach, kale, Swiss chard), roughly chopped
- 2 cloves garlic, minced
- Salt and black pepper to taste
- 1/4 cup grated Parmesan cheese (optional)
- Fresh parsley, for garnish

Instructions:

Prepare the Polenta: In a medium saucepan, bring the vegetable broth or water to a boil. Gradually whisk in the polenta, reducing the heat to low. Cook, stirring frequently, until the polenta thickens and becomes creamy (about 20-25 minutes). Remove from heat and season with a pinch of salt.

Sauté the Greens: While the polenta is cooking, heat the olive oil in a large skillet over medium heat. Add the minced garlic and sauté for 1-2 minutes until fragrant. Add the mixed greens and cook, stirring occasionally, until they are wilted and tender. Season with salt and black pepper.

Serve: Spoon the creamy polenta onto plates or bowls, top with the sautéed greens, and sprinkle with grated Parmesan cheese (if using). Garnish with fresh parsley.

Nutritional Data: Calories: 210 | Total Fat: 5g | Saturated Fat: 1g | Cholesterol: 5mg | Sodium: 150mg | Total Carbohydrates: 34g | Dietary Fiber: 4g | Sugars: 1g | Protein: 7g

Roasted Vegetable Platter

Preparation Time: 20 minutes | Cooking Time: 40 minutes | Portion Size: 6 servings

Ingredients:
- 2 medium zucchinis, sliced into half-moons
- 1 large red bell pepper, cut into strips
- 1 large yellow bell pepper, cut into strips
- 2 medium carrots, sliced diagonally
- 1 cup green beans, trimmed
- 1 cup Brussels sprouts, halved
- 3 tablespoons olive oil
- Salt to taste
- 1 tablespoon fresh thyme leaves
- 1 tablespoon fresh rosemary, finely chopped

Instructions:

Preheat the Oven: Preheat your oven to 400°F (200°C).

Prepare the Vegetables: Wash and slice all the vegetables as mentioned in the ingredients list.

Toss the Vegetables: In a large mixing bowl, toss the vegetables with olive oil, salt, thyme, and rosemary. Ensure all the pieces are well-coated with the oil and herbs.

Roasting: Spread the seasoned vegetables in a single layer on a large baking sheet. Make sure they are not overcrowded; use two sheets if necessary.

Bake: Place the baking sheet(s) in the oven and roast the vegetables for about 35-40 minutes, or until they are tender and slightly golden. Turn the vegetables halfway through the roasting time to ensure even cooking.

Serve: Once done, remove from the oven and transfer the roasted vegetables to a serving platter. Serve warm.

Nutritional Data: Calories: 120 | Total Fat: 7g | Saturated Fat: 1g | Cholesterol: 0mg | Sodium: 60mg | Total Carbohydrates: 14g | Dietary Fiber: 5g | Sugars: 6g | Protein: 3g

Tuna & Avocado Salad

Preparation Time: 15 minutes | Portion Size: 4 servings

Ingredients:
- 2 cans (5 oz each) solid white tuna in water, drained and flaked
- 2 ripe avocados, pitted, peeled, and diced
- 1 medium cucumber, diced
- 1/4 cup red onion, finely chopped
- 1/4 cup fresh cilantro, finely chopped
- 1 tablespoon fresh lemon juice
- 2 tablespoons olive oil
- Salt and pepper to taste
- 2 cups mixed salad greens (like spinach, arugula, and romaine)

Instructions:

Prepare the Ingredients: Begin by draining the tuna and flaking it into a large mixing bowl. Chop and dice the remaining ingredients as specified. Assemble the Salad: Add the diced avocados, cucumber, red onion, and cilantro to the bowl with the tuna. Dress the Salad: In a small bowl, whisk together the fresh lemon juice, olive oil, salt, and pepper. Drizzle this dressing over the tuna and vegetable mixture. Toss gently to ensure the salad is well-coated with the dressing. Serve: Lay out the mixed salad greens on individual plates or a large serving platter. Top with the tuna and avocado mixture. Serve immediately.

Nutritional Data: Calories: 270 | Total Fat: 18g | Saturated Fat: 2.5g | Cholesterol: 30mg | Sodium: 290mg | Total Carbohydrates: 12g | Dietary Fiber: 7g | Sugars: 2g | Protein: 20g

Pea & Mint Risotto

Preparation Time: 10 minutes | Cooking Time: 25 minutes | Portion Size: 4 servings

Ingredients:
- 1 cup Arborio rice
- 2 tablespoons olive oil
- 1 small onion, finely chopped
- 3 cloves garlic, minced
- 4 cups low-sodium vegetable broth, warmed
- 2 cups fresh or frozen peas
- 1/2 cup fresh mint leaves, finely chopped
- Zest and juice of 1 lemon
- 1/4 cup grated Parmesan cheese (optional)
- Salt and pepper to taste

Instructions:

Sauté Base Ingredients: In a large skillet or saucepan, heat the olive oil over medium heat. Add the chopped onion and minced garlic, sautéing until they're soft and translucent, which should take about 3-4 minutes.

Cook the Rice: Stir in the Arborio rice, ensuring it's well-coated in the olive oil. Cook for 1-2 minutes, or until the rice has a slight translucent edge. Begin adding the warmed vegetable broth one ladle at a time, stirring frequently. Wait until most of the liquid is absorbed before adding the next ladle of broth.

Add the Peas: When the rice is about halfway cooked (after about 12-15 minutes), stir in the peas. Continue to add broth and stir the risotto.

Final Touches: Once the rice is tender and the risotto has a creamy consistency, stir in the chopped mint, lemon zest, lemon juice, and grated Parmesan cheese if using. Season with salt and pepper to taste.

Serve: Serve the risotto immediately, garnishing with extra mint leaves or a sprinkle of Parmesan if desired.

Nutritional Data: Calories: 340 | Total Fat: 8g | Saturated Fat: 1.5g | Cholesterol: 5mg | Sodium: 150mg | Total Carbohydrates: 58g | Dietary Fiber: 4g | Sugars: 5g | Protein: 9g

Loaded Sweet Potato

Preparation Time: 15 minutes | Cooking Time: 45 minutes | Portion Size: 4 servings

---

Ingredients:
- 4 medium-sized sweet potatoes
- 2 tablespoons olive oil
- 1 cup cooked quinoa
- 1/2 cup black beans, rinsed and drained
- 1 avocado, sliced
- 1/2 cup Greek yogurt (or non-dairy alternative)
- 2 green onions, finely sliced
- Salt and pepper to taste
- Fresh cilantro (optional) for garnish

Instructions:

Preheat and Prep: Preheat your oven to 400°F (200°C). While waiting, wash and scrub the sweet potatoes thoroughly. Pat them dry using a clean towel.

Roast Sweet Potatoes: Prick the sweet potatoes all over with a fork. Lightly coat them with olive oil and place them on a baking sheet. Roast in the preheated oven for 40-45 minutes or until they are tender and can be easily pierced with a fork.

Prepare Toppings: While the sweet potatoes are baking, prepare the quinoa according to its package instructions, if not already cooked. Set aside. In a separate bowl, mix the black beans, salt, and pepper. Slice the avocado and green onions.

Assemble: Once the sweet potatoes are done, remove them from the oven and let them cool slightly. Carefully slice each potato open lengthwise, and fluff the insides with a fork. Stuff each sweet potato with a generous portion of quinoa and black beans. Top with avocado slices and a dollop of Greek yogurt.

Serve: Garnish with green onions and cilantro if desired. Serve immediately while warm.

Nutritional Data: Calories: 320 | Total Fat: 10g | Saturated Fat: 2g | Cholesterol: 3mg | Sodium: 105mg | Total Carbohydrates: 50g | Dietary Fiber: 9g | Sugars: 8g | Protein: 8g

Silky Sesame & Chicken Cold Noodles

Preparation Time: 20 minutes | Cooking Time: 20 minutes | Portion Size: 4 servings

Ingredients:

- 8 oz (about 225g) flat rice noodles or soba noodles
- 2 boneless, skinless chicken breasts
- 2 tablespoons toasted sesame oil
- 3 tablespoons low-sodium soy sauce (or tamari for gluten-free)
- 1 tablespoon rice vinegar
- 1 teaspoon honey or maple syrup
- 2 green onions, finely sliced
- 1 tablespoon sesame seeds (white or black)
- 1 cup thinly sliced cucumber
- 1 red bell pepper, thinly sliced
- Salt to taste
- Fresh cilantro leaves for garnish (optional)

Instructions:

Cook Noodles: In a large pot of boiling water, cook the noodles according to the package instructions until al dente. Once cooked, drain and rinse under cold water to cool them down. Set aside. Cook Chicken: Season chicken breasts lightly with salt. In a skillet over medium heat, cook the chicken until fully cooked through, about 7 minutes per side depending on thickness. Once cooked, remove from heat, let it cool, then shred the chicken using two forks. Prepare Sesame Sauce: In a mixing bowl, whisk together toasted sesame oil, low-sodium soy sauce, rice vinegar, and honey or maple syrup until well combined. Combine and Toss: In a large mixing bowl, combine the cold noodles, shredded chicken, sliced cucumber, and red bell pepper. Drizzle with the sesame sauce and toss to ensure everything is well-coated. Divide the noodle mixture among plates or bowls. Garnish with green onions, sesame seeds, and cilantro if desired. Serve cold.

Nutritional Data: Calories: 315 | Total Fat: 9g | Saturated Fat: 1.5g | Cholesterol: 55mg | Sodium: 320mg | Total Carbohydrates: 38g | Dietary Fiber: 2g | Sugars: 4g | Protein: 22g

Beet & Barley Bowl with Lemon Zest

Preparation Time: 15 minutes | Cooking Time: 40 minutes | Portion Size: 4 servings

Ingredients:

- 1 cup pearl barley, rinsed
- 3 cups water or low-sodium vegetable broth
- 3 medium golden beets, peeled and diced
- 2 tablespoons olive oil
- Zest of 1 lemon
- 1 tablespoon lemon juice
- 1/4 cup fresh parsley, chopped
- 1/4 cup toasted walnuts, chopped
- 1/4 cup crumbled feta cheese (optional)
- Freshly ground black pepper

Instructions:

In a medium saucepan, bring the water or vegetable broth to a boil. Add the barley and a pinch of salt. Reduce the heat, cover, and simmer for 30-35 minutes or until the barley is tender. Drain any excess liquid and set aside. While the barley is cooking, preheat the oven to 400°F (200°C). Toss the diced golden beets in 1 tablespoon of olive oil and spread them on a baking sheet. Season lightly with salt. Roast in the oven for 20-25 minutes or until tender and slightly golden. Prepare Lemon Zest Dressing: In a small bowl, whisk together the remaining 1 tablespoon of olive oil, lemon zest, and lemon juice. Assemble the Bowl: In a large mixing bowl, combine the cooked barley, roasted golden beets, and fresh parsley. Drizzle with the lemon zest dressing and toss to combine. Divide the barley and beet mixture among bowls. Top each bowl with toasted walnuts, crumbled feta cheese (if using), and a sprinkle of freshly ground black pepper. Serve warm or at room temperature.

Nutritional Data: Calories: 270 | Total Fat: 10g | Saturated Fat: 2g | Cholesterol: 5mg (if using feta) | Sodium: 200mg | Total Carbohydrates: 40g | Dietary Fiber: 8g | Sugars: 5g | Protein: 7g

Chapter 6: Dinner

Dinner is a cherished ritual, far more than just the final meal of the day. It represents the culmination of our daily journey, a moment for reflection and gratitude, and often a shared experience with our cherished loved ones. It encapsulates the comforting embrace of a well-prepared meal at the end of a tiring day, the sheer delight of diverse flavors dancing on our taste buds, and the sheer satisfaction of wholesome nourishment.

However, for those grappling with the discomfort of acid reflux, dinner can sometimes be approached with trepidation. Questions may arise - which foods might trigger that familiar discomfort? Can the richness of flavor be maintained without inviting the repercussions of indigestion?

In the illuminating chapter on "Dinner Recipes," we aim to unravel a treasure trove of culinary creations meticulously crafted with the twin objectives of taste and tenderness. Within these pages, you'll discover a handpicked selection of recipes that promise the joys of a hearty dinner without the nagging worry of acid reflux. Each recipe is a testament to the fact that dinner can be both a delightful and gentle experience.

These dishes have been thoughtfully designed to minimize the risk of acid reflux discomfort while maximizing the pleasure of every bite. With these recipes, you can eagerly anticipate your evening meal, knowing that it holds the promise of culinary joy, togetherness, and the comforting assurance that flavor and tranquility can indeed coexist harmoniously.

Recipes

Lettuce Wrap with Chicken and Avocado

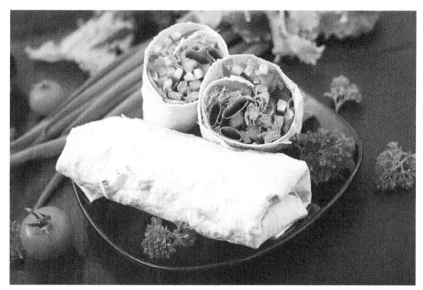

Preparation Time: 10 minutes | Cooking Time: 15 minutes | Portion Size: 4 servings

Ingredients:

- 2 boneless, skinless chicken breasts
- 1 tbsp olive oil
- 1 tsp dried oregano
- Salt and pepper, to taste
- 1 large avocado, diced
- 1 small cucumber, diced
- 1 tbsp lemon juice (optional, for those who tolerate it)
- 8 large lettuce leaves (such as romaine or butter lettuce)
- Fresh parsley for garnish (optional)

Instructions:

Heat the olive oil in a skillet over medium heat. Season the chicken breasts with oregano, salt, and pepper.
Cook the chicken for about 6-7 minutes on each side, or until fully cooked. Remove from the skillet and let rest for 5 minutes, then slice thinly. In a bowl, combine the diced avocado, cucumber, and lemon juice (if using). Toss gently. Lay out the lettuce leaves and place a few slices of chicken in each leaf. Top with the avocado and cucumber mixture.
Garnish with fresh parsley if desired. Serve immediately, wrapping the lettuce around the filling to eat.

Nutritional Data:

Calories: 250 | Total Fat: 14g | Saturated Fat: 2g | Cholesterol: 55mg | Sodium: 100mg | Total Carbohydrates: 10g | Dietary Fiber: 5g | Sugars: 2g | Protein: 22g

Barley Risotto with Zucchini and Parsley

Preparation Time: 10 minutes | Cooking Time: 35 minutes | Portion Size: 4 servings

Ingredients:
- 1 cup pearl barley
- 1 tbsp olive oil
- 1 small onion, finely chopped (optional, or use leek for a milder option)
- 2 medium zucchinis, diced
- 4 cups low-sodium vegetable broth
- 1/4 cup fresh parsley, chopped
- 1 tsp dried thyme
- 2 tbsp grated Parmesan cheese (optional, for garnish)

Instructions:

Heat the olive oil in a large saucepan over medium heat. If using onion, sauté it for about 5 minutes until soft. Add the pearl barley and stir to coat in the oil. Cook for 2-3 minutes until lightly toasted. Gradually add the vegetable broth, one cup at a time, stirring frequently and allowing the liquid to absorb before adding more. Continue this process for about 30 minutes, until the barley is tender and creamy. In the last 10 minutes of cooking, stir in the diced zucchini and thyme, allowing the zucchini to cook until tender. Once the barley is cooked, stir in the fresh parsley and season with salt and pepper to taste. Serve the risotto hot, optionally garnished with grated Parmesan cheese.

Nutritional Data:

Calories: 260 | Total Fat: 6g | Saturated Fat: 1g | Cholesterol: 0mg | Sodium: 250mg | Total Carbohydrates: 45g | Dietary Fiber: 8g | Sugars: 4g | Protein: 8g

Grilled Tilapia with Herbed Quinoa

Preparation Time: 20 minutes | Cooking Time: 15 minutes | Portion Size: 4 servings

Ingredients:
- 4 tilapia fillets
- 1 cup quinoa, rinsed and drained
- 2 cups low-sodium vegetable broth
- 1 tablespoon olive oil
- 2 garlic cloves, minced
- Zest and juice of 1 lemon
- 1/4 cup fresh parsley, finely chopped
- 1/4 cup fresh chives, finely chopped
- Salt to taste
- Freshly ground black pepper
- Olive oil spray or brush for grilling

Instructions:

To prepare the quinoa, scald the vegetable broth in a medium pot. When all the liquid has been absorbed, add the quinoa, lower the heat to low, cover, and simmer for 15 minutes. After 5 minutes of cooling, remove from heat and fluff with a fork.

Quinoa with Herbs: In a different skillet, warm the olive oil over medium heat. For one to two minutes, add the garlic and sauté. Add the parsley, chives, lemon zest, and juice after turning off the heat. Add salt and pepper to taste and combine with the cooked quinoa.

Tilapia grilling instructions: Heat the grill or grill pan to medium. Salt and pepper the tilapia fillets just enough to give them flavour. Apply some mist or a little brushing.

Nutritional Data: Calories: 280 | Total Fat: 6g | Saturated Fat: 1g | Cholesterol: 55mg | Sodium: 150mg | Total Carbohydrates: 30g | Dietary Fiber: 3g | Sugars: 1g | Protein: 28g

Butternut & Barley Risotto

Preparation Time: 20 minutes | Cooking Time: 45 minutes | Portion Size: 4 servings

Ingredients:

- 1 cup pearled barley, rinsed
- 3 cups butternut squash, diced
- 4 cups low-sodium vegetable broth
- 1 small onion, finely chopped
- 2 garlic cloves, minced
- 1 tablespoon olive oil
- 1/4 cup fresh parsley, chopped
- Salt to taste
- Freshly ground black pepper
- 1/4 cup grated Parmesan cheese (optional)
- 1/4 cup unsweetened almond milk

Instructions:

Sauté Base: In a large pot, heat the olive oil over medium heat. Add the chopped onions and sauté until translucent, about 5 minutes. Add the minced garlic and sauté for another 1-2 minutes. Cook Barley: Stir in the pearled barley, ensuring it's well-coated with the oil and onion mixture. Cook for 2 minutes, stirring frequently. Risotto Process: Begin adding the vegetable broth, half a cup at a time, allowing each addition to be mostly absorbed before adding more. Stir frequently to prevent sticking. Butternut Squash: After you've added about half of the broth, stir in the diced butternut squash. Continue with the risotto cooking process, adding the remaining broth bit by bit. Finishing Touches: Once the barley is tender and the butternut squash is soft (about 40 minutes in total), reduce the heat to low. Stir in the almond milk, parsley, and grated Parmesan cheese if desired. Season with salt and pepper to taste. Dish out the risotto into bowls and garnish with a bit more parsley or Parmesan if desired. Enjoy your dusk delight!

Nutritional Data: Calories: 320 | Total Fat: 6g | Saturated Fat: 1.5g | Cholesterol: 5mg (if using Parmesan) | Sodium: 200mg | Total Carbohydrates: 58g | Dietary Fiber: 10g | Sugars: 4g | Protein: 9g

Tofu Stir-Fry with Veggies

Preparation Time: 15 minutes | Cooking Time: 20 minutes | Portion Size: 4 servings

Ingredients:
- 1 block (14 oz) firm tofu, drained, pressed, and cubed
- 2 cups broccoli florets
- 1 red bell pepper, sliced
- 1 carrot, julienned
- 2 green onions, sliced
- 2 tablespoons olive oil
- 2 tablespoons low-sodium soy sauce (or tamari for gluten-free option)
- 1 tablespoon ginger, grated
- 1 tablespoon toasted sesame oil
- 2 garlic cloves, minced
- 1 tablespoon cornstarch (mixed with 2 tablespoons water)
- Salt to taste
- Freshly ground black pepper

Instructions:

Prep Tofu: After draining and pressing the tofu, cut it into bite-sized cubes. Set aside. Stir-Fry Base: In a large skillet or wok, heat the olive oil over medium-high heat. Once hot, add the tofu cubes, letting them cook until golden on each side, about 4-5 minutes total. Veggies Time: Add the broccoli florets, sliced bell pepper, and julienned carrot to the skillet. Stir-fry for another 5-7 minutes, or until the veggies are just tender but still retain a crisp bite. Flavor Burst: In a separate bowl, combine the low-sodium soy sauce, grated ginger, minced garlic, and toasted sesame oil. Mix well and pour the sauce mixture over the tofu and veggies in the skillet. Once the sauce starts to sizzle, quickly stir in the cornstarch mixture. Stir continuously until the sauce thickens, coating the tofu and veggies evenly. Season with salt and pepper as needed. Stir in the sliced green onions just before removing from the heat.

Nutritional Data: Calories: 220 | Total Fat: 12g | Saturated Fat: 2g | Cholesterol: 0mg | Sodium: 320mg | Total Carbohydrates: 15g | Dietary Fiber: 3g | Sugars: 4g | Protein: 14g

Soothing Spaghetti Squash with Olive Tapenade

Preparation Time: 15 minutes | Cooking Time: 40 minutes | Portion Size: 4 servings

Ingredients:
- 1 medium spaghetti squash (about 2-3 pounds)
- 1 cup pitted Kalamata olives
- 1 cup pitted green olives
- 2 tablespoons capers, drained
- 2 garlic cloves, minced
- 1/4 cup extra-virgin olive oil
- 1 tablespoon lemon juice
- 2 tablespoons fresh parsley, chopped
- Salt to taste
- Freshly ground black pepper

Instructions:

Cook the Spaghetti Squash: Preheat your oven to 400°F (200°C). Cut the spaghetti squash in half lengthwise and scoop out the seeds. Place the halves face-down on a baking sheet and roast in the oven for about 35-40 minutes, or until the flesh easily shreds with a fork. Once cooked, use a fork to scrape out the "spaghetti" strands from the squash and transfer to a serving dish.

Prepare the Tapenade: While the squash is roasting, combine the Kalamata olives, green olives, capers, minced garlic, olive oil, and lemon juice in a food processor. Pulse until the mixture becomes a coarse paste. If needed, add more olive oil for a smoother texture.

Seasoning: Mix in the fresh parsley and season with salt and black pepper. Remember, olives and capers can be quite salty, so taste the tapenade before adding any additional salt.

Serve: Top the spaghetti squash strands with the olive tapenade. Toss gently to combine if desired, or leave as a topping for each individual to mix as they please.

Garnish (Optional): Sprinkle with some additional chopped parsley or a drizzle of olive oil before serving.

Nutritional Data: Calories: 220 | Total Fat: 16g | Saturated Fat: 2g | Cholesterol: 0mg | Sodium: 600mg | Total Carbohydrates: 20g | Dietary Fiber: 4g | Sugars: 7g | Protein: 2g

Herb-Infused Chicken Breast

Preparation Time: 10 minutes | Cooking Time: 25 minutes | Portion Size: 4 servings

Ingredients:

- 4 boneless, skinless chicken breasts
- 2 tablespoons olive oil
- 2 cloves garlic, minced
- 1 teaspoon fresh rosemary, finely chopped
- 1 teaspoon fresh thyme, finely chopped
- 1 teaspoon fresh parsley, finely chopped
- Salt to taste
- Freshly ground black pepper
- 1/2 cup low-sodium chicken broth

Instructions:

Herb Mixture: In a small bowl, combine the minced garlic, chopped rosemary, thyme, parsley, salt, and black pepper.

Chicken Prep: Lightly season the chicken breasts with salt and pepper. Then rub the herb mixture onto both sides of each chicken breast, ensuring they are well coated.

Cooking: In a large skillet, heat the olive oil over medium heat. Once hot, add the chicken breasts. Cook each side for about 5-7 minutes or until they begin to turn golden brown.

Simmer: After the chicken is browned, pour the low-sodium chicken broth into the skillet. Let it come to a simmer, then reduce the heat to low. Cover and let the chicken cook for another 10-12 minutes, or until fully cooked through.

Serve: Once cooked, transfer the chicken breasts to a serving plate. You can drizzle a little of the remaining broth from the skillet over the top for added moisture and flavor.

Nutritional Data: Calories: 210 | Total Fat: 8g | Saturated Fat: 1.5g | Cholesterol: 85mg | Sodium: 150mg | Total Carbohydrates: 1g | Dietary Fiber: 0g | Sugars: 0g | Protein: 30g

Fennel & White Bean Stew

Preparation Time: 15 minutes | Cooking Time: 20 minutes | Portion Size: 4 servings

Ingredients:

- 2 fennel bulbs, thinly sliced
- 2 cans (15 oz each) white beans, rinsed and drained
- 2 tablespoons olive oil
- 1 onion, finely chopped
- 3 cloves garlic, minced
- 4 cups vegetable broth, low-sodium
- 1 teaspoon fresh thyme leaves
- 1 bay leaf
- Salt to taste
- Freshly ground black pepper
- 2 tablespoons fresh parsley, chopped (for garnish)
- Zest of 1 lemon (optional for added zing)

Instructions:

Sauté Basics: In a large pot or Dutch oven, heat the olive oil over medium heat. Add the chopped onions and sauté until translucent, about 3-4 minutes. Add the garlic and fennel slices, continuing to sauté for another 5 minutes, or until the fennel begins to soften. Beans & Broth: Stir in the white beans, followed by the vegetable broth. Mix everything well, ensuring the ingredients are well-combined. Herbs & Seasoning: Add the fresh thyme leaves and bay leaf to the pot. Season with salt and freshly ground black pepper. Mix well. Simmer: Reduce the heat to low and let the stew simmer for about 10-12 minutes, allowing the flavors to meld. Finishing Touches: Just before serving, remove the bay leaf and stir in the fresh parsley and lemon zest if desired. Ladle the stew into bowls and serve warm.

Nutritional Data: Calories: 250 | Total Fat: 7g | Saturated Fat: 1g | Cholesterol: 0mg | Sodium: 300mg | Total Carbohydrates: 38g | Dietary Fiber: 10g | Sugars: 3g | Protein: 12g

Mushroom & Brown Rice Bowl

Preparation Time: 20 minutes | Cooking Time: 45 minutes (includes rice cooking time) | Portion Size: 4 servings

Ingredients:

- 1 cup brown rice, rinsed and drained
- 2.5 cups water
- 2 tablespoons olive oil
- 1 onion, finely chopped
- 3 cloves garlic, minced
- 2 cups assorted mushrooms (like cremini, shiitake, and button), sliced
- 1/2 cup low-sodium vegetable broth
- 2 tablespoons fresh parsley, chopped
- Salt to taste
- Freshly ground black pepper
- 1/4 cup toasted almond slices (for garnish)
- 1 green onion, thinly sliced (for garnish)

Instructions:

Rice Preparation: In a saucepan, bring the water to a boil. Add the brown rice, reduce the heat to low, cover, and let simmer for about 35-40 minutes, or until the rice is cooked and all the water is absorbed. Remove from heat and set aside.

Mushroom Sauté: While the rice is cooking, heat olive oil in a large skillet over medium heat. Add the chopped onions and sauté until translucent. Introduce the minced garlic and sauté for an additional minute, until aromatic.

Mushroom Medley: Add the assorted sliced mushrooms to the skillet. Cook, occasionally stirring, until the mushrooms release their moisture and begin to brown slightly, about 8-10 minutes. Broth & Season: Pour in the vegetable broth to deglaze the skillet, scraping up any browned bits from the bottom. Allow the mixture to simmer for 5-7 minutes, or until slightly reduced. Season with salt and freshly ground black pepper.

Combine & Serve: Divide the cooked brown rice among four bowls. Top each bowl with an equal portion of the mushroom mixture. Garnish with toasted almond slices, fresh parsley, and sliced green onions.

Nutritional Data: Calories: 280 | Total Fat: 9g | Saturated Fat: 1.5g | Cholesterol: 0mg | Sodium: 150mg | Total Carbohydrates: 44g | Dietary Fiber: 4g | Sugars: 2g | Protein: 7g

Lemon-Poached Cod with Spinach

Preparation Time: 10 minutes | Cooking Time: 20 minutes | Portion Size: 4 servings

Ingredients:

- 4 cod fillets (approximately 6 oz. each)
- Zest and juice of 2 lemons
- 2 cups low-sodium vegetable broth
- 2 tablespoons olive oil
- 4 cloves garlic, minced
- 8 cups fresh spinach, washed and roughly chopped
- Salt to taste
- Freshly ground black pepper
- 1 tablespoon fresh dill, chopped (for garnish)
- Lemon slices, for serving

Instructions:

Prepare Cod: Ensure cod fillets are cleaned and free of bones. Set aside.

Lemon-Poaching: In a large skillet or shallow saucepan, combine the lemon zest, lemon juice, and vegetable broth. Bring to a gentle simmer over medium heat.

Poach the Cod: Gently add the cod fillets to the simmering broth. Cover and let the fish poach for about 10-12 minutes, or until the cod becomes opaque and flakes easily with a fork.

Spinach Sauté: While the cod is poaching, in another skillet, heat olive oil over medium heat. Add the minced garlic and sauté until aromatic, about 1 minute. Introduce the chopped spinach and cook until just wilted, about 2-3 minutes. Season lightly with salt and black pepper.

Serve: Place a portion of the wilted spinach on each plate. Carefully lift the poached cod fillets from the broth and place them atop the spinach. Garnish with fresh dill and serve with a slice of lemon on the side.

Nutritional Data: Calories: 220 | Total Fat: 8g | Saturated Fat: 1.2g | Cholesterol: 60mg | Sodium: 180mg | Total Carbohydrates: 6g | Dietary Fiber: 2g | Sugars: 1g | Protein: 30g

Chickpea and Sweet Potato Patties

Preparation Time: 15 minutes | Cooking Time: 30 minutes | Portion Size: 4 servings

Ingredients:

- 1 medium sweet potato, peeled and diced
- 1 (15 oz) can chickpeas, drained and rinsed
- 1/2 cup breadcrumbs (whole wheat or gluten-free)
- 1 egg, lightly beaten
- 1 tbsp olive oil
- 1 tsp dried oregano
- 1 tsp cumin
- Salt and pepper, to taste
- Fresh parsley, chopped (optional, for garnish)

Instructions:

Preheat the oven to 375°F (190°C) and line a baking sheet with parchment paper. Boil the sweet potato in a pot of water for about 10-12 minutes, or until soft. Drain and mash with a fork. In a large bowl, combine the mashed sweet potato, chickpeas, breadcrumbs, beaten egg, olive oil, oregano, cumin, salt, and pepper. Mash the chickpeas slightly to help the mixture stick together. Form the mixture into small patties and place them on the prepared baking sheet. Bake for 20-25 minutes, flipping halfway through, until golden brown and firm. Garnish with fresh parsley if desired, and serve warm.

Nutritional Data:
Calories: 220 | Total Fat: 7g | Saturated Fat: 1g | Cholesterol: 40mg | Sodium: 180mg | Total Carbohydrates: 35g | Dietary Fiber: 7g | Sugars: 6g | Protein: 7g

Eggplant & Chickpea Curry

Preparation Time: 15 minutes | Cooking Time: 30 minutes | Portion Size: 4 servings

Ingredients:
- 2 medium eggplants, cubed
- 1 can (15 oz) chickpeas, drained and rinsed
- 1 onion, finely chopped
- 2 cloves garlic, minced
- 1-inch ginger, grated
- 1 tablespoon coconut oil
- 1 can (13.5 oz) light coconut milk
- 2 teaspoons ground turmeric
- 1 teaspoon ground cumin
- 1/2 teaspoon ground coriander
- Fresh cilantro, chopped (for garnish)
- Cooked brown rice or quinoa (for serving)

Instructions:

In a large pot or skillet, heat the coconut oil over medium heat. Add the onion, garlic, and ginger. Sauté until the onion is translucent and aromatic. Stir in the ground turmeric, cumin, and coriander. Cook for an additional 1-2 minutes until the spices release their aromas. Add the cubed eggplant to the pot, ensuring they're well-coated with the onion-spice mixture. Cook for about 10 minutes, or until the eggplant starts to soften. Pour in the coconut milk and chickpeas. Mix well and let the curry simmer for another 15 minutes, stirring occasionally. If the curry appears too thick, you can add a bit of water to reach the desired consistency. Season the curry with salt, adjusting to taste. Serve the curry hot over cooked brown rice or quinoa. Garnish with fresh cilantro.

Nutritional Data: Calories: 260 | Total Fat: 10g | Saturated Fat: 7g | Cholesterol: 0mg | Sodium: 300mg | Total Carbohydrates: 36g | Dietary Fiber: 10g | Sugars: 9g | Protein: 8g

Steamed Veggies & Pesto

Preparation Time: 10 minutes | Cooking Time: 15 minutes | Portion Size: 4 servings

Ingredients:

- 2 cups broccoli florets
- 2 cups cauliflower florets
- 1 cup sliced carrots
- 1 cup green beans, trimmed
- 1/2 cup fresh basil leaves
- 1/4 cup pine nuts
- 2 cloves garlic
- 1/4 cup grated Parmesan cheese (optional)
- 1/4 cup extra-virgin olive oil
- Salt and pepper, to taste

Instructions:

In a steamer or a pot with a steaming basket, bring about an inch of water to a boil. Place the broccoli, cauliflower, carrots, and green beans in the steaming basket. Cover and steam the veggies for about 10-12 minutes or until they are tender but still have a bit of a bite. While the veggies are steaming, prepare the pesto. In a food processor or blender, combine the fresh basil, pine nuts, garlic, and grated Parmesan cheese (if using). Process until finely chopped. With the processor running, drizzle in the olive oil until a smooth paste forms. Season the pesto with salt and pepper according to your taste. Once the vegetables are steamed, transfer them to a serving dish. Drizzle the pesto over the veggies or serve it on the side. Toss the veggies with the pesto until they're well coated.

Nutritional Data: Calories: 220 | Total Fat: 18g | Saturated Fat: 3g | Cholesterol: 5mg | Sodium: 180mg | Total Carbohydrates: 12g | Dietary Fiber: 4g | Sugars: 4g | Protein: 6g

Baked Falafel with Tzatziki

Preparation Time: 20 minutes | Cooking Time: 30 minutes | Portion Size: 4 servings

Ingredients:
For the Baked Falafel:
- 2 cups canned chickpeas, rinsed and drained
- 1/4 cup fresh parsley, chopped
- 1/4 cup fresh cilantro, chopped
- 3 cloves garlic, minced
- 1 tsp ground cumin
- 1/2 tsp ground coriander
- Salt and pepper, to taste
- 2 tbsp olive oil
- 1 tsp baking powder

For the Tzatziki:
- 1 cup Greek yogurt (or a dairy-free alternative)
- 1/2 cucumber, seeded and finely diced
- 2 cloves garlic, minced
- 1 tbsp lemon juice
- 1 tbsp fresh dill, chopped
- Salt and pepper, to taste

Instructions:

Falafel: In a food processor, combine the chickpeas, parsley, cilantro, garlic, cumin, coriander, salt, and pepper. Process until almost smooth but still a little chunky.

Transfer the mixture to a bowl and stir in the baking powder.

Preheat the oven to 375°F (190°C). Line a baking sheet with parchment paper.

Shape the falafel mixture into small balls or patties and place them on the prepared baking sheet. Drizzle or brush them with olive oil.

Bake in the preheated oven for 25-30 minutes or until golden and crispy on the outside.

Tzatziki: While the falafel bakes, prepare the tzatziki. In a bowl, combine the Greek yogurt, cucumber, garlic, lemon juice, and dill. Season with salt and pepper to taste. Mix well.

Serve the baked falafel warm with the tzatziki sauce on the side.

Nutritional Data: Calories: 280 | Total Fat: 11g | Saturated Fat: 2g | Cholesterol: 5mg | Sodium: 300mg | Total Carbohydrates: 32g | Dietary Fiber: 8g | Sugars: 6g | Protein: 12g

Quiche with Spinach & Feta

Preparation Time: 15 minutes | Cooking Time: 40 minutes | Portion Size: 8 servings

Ingredients:
For the Crust:
- 1 1/2 cups whole wheat flour
- 1/2 cup cold unsalted butter, cubed
- 1/4 cup cold water
- Pinch of salt

For the Filling:
- 2 cups fresh spinach, washed and chopped
- 1 cup feta cheese, crumbled
- 4 large eggs
- 1 1/4 cups milk (or unsweetened almond milk)
- 1/2 tsp black pepper
- 1/4 tsp nutmeg
- Salt, to taste

Instructions:

Crust: In a large mixing bowl, combine the whole wheat flour and salt. Using your fingertips or a pastry blender, incorporate the cold butter cubes until the mixture resembles coarse breadcrumbs. Gradually add the cold water, mixing until the dough comes together. Flatten the dough into a disc, wrap in plastic wrap, and refrigerate for at least 30 minutes.

Preheat your oven to 375°F (190°C).

Roll out the dough on a floured surface into a circle about 12 inches in diameter. Transfer to a 9-inch pie dish, trimming any excess and crimping the edges.

Filling: In a medium-sized skillet over medium heat, sauté the spinach until wilted. Remove from heat and set aside.

In a separate bowl, whisk together the eggs, milk, pepper, nutmeg, and salt. Stir in the wilted spinach and crumbled feta cheese.

Pour the filling into the prepared crust.

Bake in the preheated oven for 35-40 minutes, or until the quiche is set and the top is lightly golden.

Allow the quiche to cool slightly before slicing and serving.

Nutritional Data: Calories: 275 | Total Fat: 16g | Saturated Fat: 8g | Cholesterol: 115mg | Sodium: 320mg | Total Carbohydrates: 21g | Dietary Fiber: 3g | Sugars: 3g | Protein: 11g

Quinoa and Roasted Root Vegetable Salad

Preparation Time: 15 minutes | Cooking Time: 30 minutes | Portion Size: 4 servings

Ingredients:

- 1 cup quinoa, rinsed
- 2 cups water
- 2 medium carrots, peeled and diced
- 1 medium sweet potato, peeled and diced
- 1 small parsnip, peeled and diced
- 2 tbsp olive oil
- 1 tsp dried thyme
- Salt and pepper, to taste

Instructions:

Preheat the oven to 400°F (200°C). Toss the diced carrots, sweet potato, and parsnip with olive oil, thyme, salt, and pepper. Spread on a baking sheet and roast for 25-30 minutes, stirring halfway through, until tender and lightly browned. While the vegetables are roasting, cook the quinoa. In a medium saucepan, bring the quinoa and water to a boil. Reduce the heat to low, cover, and simmer for about 15 minutes or until the quinoa is cooked and the water is absorbed. Fluff with a fork and set aside. Once the vegetables are done, combine them with the cooked quinoa in a large bowl.

Nutritional Data:

Calories: 270 | Total Fat: 9g | Saturated Fat: 1.5g | Cholesterol: 0mg | Sodium: 150mg | Total Carbohydrates: 40g | Dietary Fiber: 6g | Sugars: 7g | Protein: 6g

Tempeh & Broccoli in Almond Sauce

Preparation Time: 15 minutes | Cooking Time: 25 minutes | Portion Size: 4 servings

Ingredients:

- 8 oz tempeh, cubed
- 3 cups broccoli florets
- 2 tbsp olive oil
- 1/4 cup almond butter
- 1/2 cup unsweetened almond milk
- 2 cloves garlic, minced
- 1 tbsp soy sauce (low sodium)
- 1 tsp maple syrup or agave nectar
- 1 tbsp lemon juice
- 1/4 tsp ground ginger
- Salt and pepper, to taste
- 2 tbsp slivered almonds (for garnish)
- 1 tbsp fresh chopped parsley (for garnish)

Instructions:

Begin by steaming the broccoli florets for about 4-5 minutes, ensuring they remain slightly crisp. Drain and set aside. In a skillet over medium heat, add the olive oil. Once hot, add the tempeh cubes and sauté until golden brown on all sides, approximately 5-7 minutes. Remove the tempeh and set aside. In the same skillet, add the minced garlic and sauté for about a minute until fragrant. Lower the heat and add almond butter, almond milk, soy sauce, maple syrup, lemon juice, and ground ginger to the skillet. Stir well to combine and form a smooth sauce. If the sauce is too thick, you can add a bit more almond milk to reach your desired consistency. Return the sautéed tempeh and steamed broccoli to the skillet. Toss to coat with the almond sauce. Season with salt and pepper to taste. Simmer for another 5-7 minutes, allowing the flavors to meld. Serve warm, garnished with slivered almonds and chopped parsley.

Nutritional Data: Calories: 320 | Total Fat: 22g | Saturated Fat: 3g | Cholesterol: 0mg | Sodium: 250mg | Total Carbohydrates: 20g | Dietary Fiber: 5g | Sugars: 5g | Protein: 16g

Potato & Leek Soup

Preparation Time: 15 minutes | Cooking Time: 30 minutes | Portion Size: 6 servings

Ingredients:

- 4 medium-sized potatoes, peeled and diced
- 3 leeks, white and pale green parts only, cleaned and thinly sliced
- 2 tbsp olive oil
- 4 cups low-sodium vegetable broth
- 1 cup unsweetened almond milk or other plant-based milk
- 1 bay leaf
- Salt and pepper, to taste
- 1 tsp dried thyme
- 1 tbsp fresh parsley, chopped (for garnish)
- 1 tbsp chives, chopped (for garnish)

Instructions:

In a large pot, heat the olive oil over medium heat. Add the sliced leeks and sauté until they are soft and translucent, about 5-7 minutes. Add the diced potatoes, thyme, bay leaf, and vegetable broth to the pot. Bring the mixture to a boil, then reduce to a simmer. Cover and let it simmer for 20-25 minutes, or until the potatoes are tender. Remove the bay leaf and then use an immersion blender (or transfer the soup to a blender in batches) to puree the soup until smooth. Return the pot to the heat and stir in the almond milk. Season with salt and pepper to taste. Continue to cook for another 2-3 minutes until the soup is heated through. Serve hot, garnished with fresh parsley and chives.

Nutritional Data: Calories: 190 | Total Fat: 4g | Saturated Fat: 0.5g | Cholesterol: 0mg | Sodium: 170mg | Total Carbohydrates: 36g | Dietary Fiber: 4g | Sugars: 4g | Protein: 4g

Waldorf Salad

Preparation Time: 15 minutes   (No cooking required) | Portion Size: 4 servings

Ingredients:
- 2 red apples, cored and diced
- 2 celery stalks, thinly sliced
- 1/2 cup seedless red grapes, halved
- 1/2 cup walnuts, toasted and chopped
- 1/3 cup unsweetened dried cranberries or raisins
- 1/2 cup plain yogurt (preferably low-fat or non-fat)
- 1 tbsp honey or maple syrup (optional for sweetness)
- 1 tbsp lemon juice
- 1/4 tsp vanilla extract
- Pinch of salt
- Fresh mint leaves, for garnish (optional)

Instructions:

In a large bowl, combine the diced apples, sliced celery, halved grapes, chopped walnuts, and dried cranberries or raisins.

In a separate smaller bowl, whisk together the plain yogurt, honey or maple syrup (if using), lemon juice, vanilla extract, and a pinch of salt. Mix until smooth and well combined.

Pour the yogurt mixture over the fruit and nut mixture. Gently fold everything together until all the ingredients are well coated.

Chill in the refrigerator for at least 1 hour before serving to allow the flavors to meld.

Serve in individual bowls or on salad plates, garnished with fresh mint leaves if desired.

Nutritional Data: Calories: 210 | Total Fat: 9g | Saturated Fat: 1.5g | Cholesterol: 3mg | Sodium: 60mg | Total Carbohydrates: 30g | Dietary Fiber: 4g | Sugars: 23g | Protein: 4g

Savory Stuffed Acorn Squash

Preparation Time: 20 minutes | Cooking Time: 50 minutes | Portion Size: 4 servings

Ingredients:

- 2 medium acorn squashes, halved and seeds removed
- 2 tbsp olive oil
- 1/2 cup quinoa, rinsed
- 1 cup vegetable broth (low sodium)
- 1 medium onion, finely diced
- 2 cloves garlic, minced
- 1 medium carrot, diced
- 1/2 cup celery, diced
- 1/4 cup cranberries or raisins
- 1/4 cup toasted pecans or walnuts, chopped
- 1/4 tsp dried thyme
- 1/4 tsp dried sage
- Salt and pepper, to taste
- Fresh parsley, chopped (for garnish)

Instructions:

Preheat your oven to 375°F (190°C).

Brush the cut sides of the acorn squash with 1 tablespoon of olive oil. Place them cut side down on a baking sheet and roast in the preheated oven for about 30 minutes, or until they are just tender.

In a saucepan, bring the vegetable broth to a boil. Add quinoa, cover, and reduce the heat to low. Cook until the quinoa is tender and the liquid is absorbed, about 15 minutes.

In a skillet, heat the remaining 1 tablespoon of olive oil over medium heat. Add the onion, garlic, carrot, and celery, and sauté until softened, about 5 minutes.

Stir in the cooked quinoa, cranberries or raisins, toasted nuts, dried thyme, dried sage, salt, and pepper. Mix well.

Remove the acorn squash from the oven and carefully turn them over. Stuff each squash half with the quinoa mixture.

Return the stuffed squash to the oven and bake for an additional 15-20 minutes, until everything is heated through and the tops are slightly golden.

Remove from the oven and let cool slightly before serving. Garnish with fresh parsley.

Nutritional Data: Calories: 290 | Total Fat: 12g | Saturated Fat: 1.5g | Cholesterol: 0mg | Sodium: 65mg | Total Carbohydrates: 41g | Dietary Fiber: 6g | Sugars: 8g | Protein: 7g

Chapter 7: Snacks

In our busy day-to-day lives, it's often the meals in between our main courses—the little bites, the quick pick-me-ups—that can either support or sabotage our wellness journey. These snacks play a crucial role in keeping our energy levels stable and our cravings at bay. However, for those who contend with acid reflux, it becomes essential that these in-between treats not only nourish the body but also satisfy cravings without triggering discomfort.

In this thoughtfully crafted chapter, "Snack Recipes," we've assembled a collection of delightful bites that serve a dual purpose. Not only are they incredibly delicious, but they are also intentionally designed to be gentle on the digestive system. Whether you find yourself yearning for a mid-morning boost or a late-night nibble, these recipes provide the perfect balance of flavors and health benefits.

Each snack in this chapter is a testament to the idea that you don't have to compromise taste for well-being. We understand that cravings strike at all hours, and these recipes are here to ensure that you can indulge guilt-free, knowing that your digestive comfort is a top priority. So, as you delve into this section, embrace the notion that snacks can be both a source of pleasure and a means of maintaining your wellness journey, keeping you energized and free from reflux-related discomfort.

Recipes

Crackers Saltine Spread with Avocado

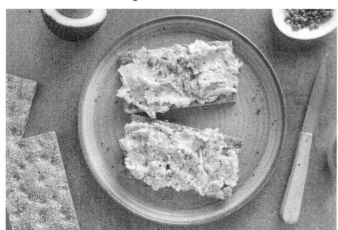

Preparation time: 10 minutes   (No cooking required) | Portion size: Makes about 1 cup (serves 4)

Ingredients:

- 2 ripe avocados, pitted and scooped
- 1/4 cup fresh cilantro, finely chopped
- 1 tablespoon fresh lime juice
- 1/4 teaspoon sea salt (adjust to taste)
- 1/4 teaspoon black pepper (optional and adjust to taste)
- 1/2 teaspoon ground flaxseed (for an added omega-3 boost)
- Saltine crackers (ensure they are low sodium for those watching salt intake)

Instructions:

In a mixing bowl, mash the avocados using a fork until they are smooth but still have some small chunks.

Add in the chopped cilantro, lime juice, sea salt, black pepper, and ground flaxseed.

Mix well until all ingredients are incorporated.

Taste and adjust seasoning if necessary.

Serve immediately with saltine crackers or store in an airtight container in the refrigerator for up to a day. If storing, place a piece of plastic wrap directly on the surface of the spread to prevent browning.

Nutritional Data: Calories: 120 per serving | Total Fat: 10g | Saturated Fat: 1.5g | Trans Fat: 0g | Cholesterol: 0mg | Sodium: 80mg | Total Carbohydrates: 7g | Dietary Fiber: 5g | Sugars: 0g | Protein: 2g

Ginger-Melon Skewers

Preparation time: 15 minutes   (No cooking required) | Portion size: Makes 12 skewers (serves 4)

Ingredients:

- 1 cup watermelon, cubed
- 1 cup honeydew melon, cubed
- 1 cup cantaloupe, cubed
- 2 tablespoons fresh ginger, finely grated
- 1 tablespoon fresh lime juice
- 1 tablespoon honey (optional)
- 12 wooden skewers

Instructions:

In a mixing bowl, combine the grated ginger, lime juice, and honey (if using). Stir well until the honey is fully dissolved. Add the melon cubes to the bowl and gently toss them in the ginger mixture, ensuring they're well coated. Thread the melon cubes onto the wooden skewers, alternating between watermelon, honeydew, and cantaloupe. Arrange the skewers on a serving platter and drizzle any remaining ginger mixture over the top. Serve immediately or refrigerate for up to 2 hours before serving. The chill will intensify the flavors and make for a refreshing snack.

Nutritional Data: Calories: 60 per skewer | Total Fat: 0.2g | Saturated Fat: 0g | Trans Fat: 0g | Cholesterol: 0mg | Sodium: 15mg | Total Carbohydrates: 15g | Dietary Fiber: 1g | Sugars: 13g | Protein: 1g

Toasted Oats & Banana Bars

Preparation time: 15 minutes | Cooking time: 25 minutes | Portion size: Makes 12 bars

Ingredients:

- 2 cups rolled oats
- 2 ripe bananas, mashed
- 1/2 cup unsweetened almond milk (or any other non-dairy milk of choice)
- 1/4 cup honey or maple syrup
- 1 teaspoon vanilla extract
- 1/2 teaspoon cinnamon
- 1/4 cup chopped walnuts (optional)
- 1/4 cup unsweetened shredded coconut
- A pinch of salt

Instructions:

Preheat the oven to 350°F (175°C) and line an 8x8-inch baking dish with parchment paper, leaving some overhang for easy removal. In a large mixing bowl, combine the mashed bananas, almond milk, honey or maple syrup, and vanilla extract. Mix until well combined. In another bowl, combine the rolled oats, cinnamon, walnuts (if using), shredded coconut, and salt. Stir to combine. Gradually add the dry ingredients to the wet mixture, stirring until just combined. Transfer the mixture to the prepared baking dish, spreading it out evenly. Bake in the preheated oven for 20-25 minutes, or until the edges are golden brown and a toothpick inserted into the center comes out mostly clean. Remove from the oven and let it cool in the pan for about 10 minutes. Using the parchment paper overhang, lift the bars out of the pan and transfer to a wire rack to cool completely. Once cooled, cut into 12 equal-sized bars.

Nutritional Data: Calories: 120 per bar | Total Fat: 3g | Saturated Fat: 1g | Trans Fat: 0g | Cholesterol: 0mg | Sodium: 25mg | Total Carbohydrates: 22g | Dietary Fiber: 3g | Sugars: 9g | Protein: 3g

Carrot & Cucumber Pinwheels

Preparation time: 15 minutes | Portion size: Makes 24 pinwheels

Ingredients:
- 4 large whole grain tortilla wraps
- 1 cup low-fat cream cheese, softened
- 1 cup finely grated carrot
- 1 cucumber, deseeded and thinly sliced lengthwise
- 2 tablespoons chopped fresh dill (or 1 tablespoon dried dill)
- A pinch of salt and black pepper

Instructions:

Lay out the tortilla wraps on a clean surface. Evenly spread the softened cream cheese across each wrap, leaving a small border around the edges. Sprinkle the grated carrot evenly over the cream cheese on each wrap. Place thin slices of cucumber on top of the carrot layer. Sprinkle the dill evenly across the cucumber and carrot layers. Season with a pinch of salt and black pepper. Starting from one end, carefully roll each tortilla into a tight roll. Using a sharp knife, slice each rolled tortilla into six even pinwheels. Serve immediately or refrigerate for later use. The pinwheels are best enjoyed the same day but can be refrigerated for up to a day.

Nutritional Data: Calories: 45 per pinwheel | Total Fat: 1.5g | Saturated Fat: 0.5g | Trans Fat: 0g | Cholesterol: 5mg | Sodium: 80mg | Total Carbohydrates: 6g | Dietary Fiber: 1g | Sugars: 1g | Protein: 2g

Mango Rice Cakes

Preparation time: 10 minutes | Portion size: Makes 6 servings

Ingredients:
- 6 plain rice cakes
- 1 ripe mango, peeled and finely diced
- 1/2 cup low-fat Greek yogurt
- 2 tablespoons honey or maple syrup (optional)
- A pinch of ground cardamom (optional)
- Fresh mint leaves for garnish

Instructions:

In a medium-sized bowl, mix the finely diced mango with honey or maple syrup and cardamom (if using) until well combined. Spread an even layer of Greek yogurt on each rice cake. Spoon a generous amount of the mango mixture onto each rice cake, spreading it out to cover the yogurt. Garnish with a mint leaf on top of each rice cake. Serve immediately for the best texture and taste.

Nutritional Data: Calories: 80 per serving | Total Fat: 0.5g | Saturated Fat: 0.2g | Trans Fat: 0g | Cholesterol: 1mg | Sodium: 30mg | Total Carbohydrates: 18g | Dietary Fiber: 1g | Sugars: 10g | Protein: 2g

Delicate Dill & Carrot Hummus

Preparation time: 10 minutes | Portion size: Makes 8 servings

Ingredients:
- 1 can (15 oz.) of chickpeas, drained and rinsed
- 2 medium carrots, peeled and finely grated
- 2 tbsp of tahini (sesame seed paste)
- Juice of 1 lemon
- 2 garlic cloves, minced (optional for those sensitive to garlic)
- 1/4 cup of fresh dill, chopped
- 2 tbsp of extra virgin olive oil
- Salt to taste
- Water as needed
- Additional dill and carrot shavings for garnish

Instructions:

In a food processor, combine the chickpeas, grated carrots, tahini, lemon juice, and minced garlic (if using). Blend until the mixture starts to become smooth. With the processor running, slowly add in the olive oil and blend until the mixture is creamy. If the hummus is too thick, you can add water, a tablespoon at a time, until you achieve the desired consistency. Fold in the chopped dill and season with salt to taste. Transfer the hummus to a serving bowl and garnish with additional dill and carrot shavings. Serve with whole grain crackers, raw vegetables, or as a spread on sandwiches.

Nutritional Data: Calories: 130 per serving | Total Fat: 5g | Saturated Fat: 0.7g | Trans Fat: 0g | Cholesterol: 0mg | Sodium: 75mg | Total Carbohydrates: 18g | Dietary Fiber: 4g | Sugars: 3g | Protein: 5g

Wheat Crackers with Tofu Dip

Preparation time: 15 minutes | Portion size: Makes 10 servings

Ingredients:
For the Tofu Dip:
- 1 cup firm tofu, drained and pressed
- 1 tbsp olive oil
- 1 tbsp fresh lemon juice
- 2 tbsp chopped fresh chives
- Salt and black pepper to taste
- 1/4 cup fresh parsley, chopped
- 1/2 tsp garlic powder (optional for those sensitive to garlic)

For Serving:
- 30 whispering wheat crackers (ensure they are low in sodium and free of any high-acidity additives)

Instructions:

Start by preparing the tofu dip. In a blender or food processor, combine the tofu, olive oil, lemon juice, chives, parsley, and garlic powder if using. Blend until smooth. Season the dip with salt and black pepper to taste. Transfer to a serving bowl. Arrange the whispering wheat crackers around the tofu dip and serve immediately.

Serving Suggestion: The tofu dip also pairs well with raw veggies like cucumber, carrot, and bell pepper sticks.

Nutritional Data: Calories: 85 per serving | Total Fat: 3g | Saturated Fat: 0.5g | Trans Fat: 0g | Cholesterol: 0mg | Sodium: 50mg | Total Carbohydrates: 10g | Dietary Fiber: 1g | Sugars: 1g | Protein: 5g

Zucchini & Parmesan Crisps

Preparation time: 10 minutes | Cooking time: 20 minutes | Portion size: Makes 4 servings

Ingredients:
- 2 medium zucchinis
- 1/2 cup grated Parmesan cheese
- 1/4 tsp black pepper
- 1/4 tsp dried oregano
- 1/4 tsp dried basil
- Olive oil spray (optional)

Instructions:

Preheat your oven to 400°F (200°C). Line a baking sheet with parchment paper or a silicone baking mat. Slice the zucchinis into thin rounds, about 1/8-inch thick. Place the zucchini slices on the baking sheet in a single layer, ensuring they do not overlap. Lightly spray the zucchini slices with olive oil. If you don't have a spray, you can lightly brush them with oil using a pastry brush. In a small bowl, mix together the grated Parmesan, black pepper, oregano, and basil. Sprinkle this mixture evenly over each zucchini slice. Bake in the preheated oven for about 15 to 20 minutes, or until the Parmesan turns a light golden brown and the zucchini slices are crisp. Remove from the oven and allow them to cool slightly before serving.

Serving Suggestion: Serve the crisps as a snack on their own or with a mild dip of choice. They are particularly delicious with a light yogurt-based dip.

Nutritional Data: Calories: 65 per serving | Total Fat: 3.5g | Saturated Fat: 2g | Trans Fat: 0g | Cholesterol: 10mg | Sodium: 160mg | Total Carbohydrates: 3g | Dietary Fiber: 1g | Sugars: 2g | Protein: 5g

Coconut and Sunflower Seed Energy Bars

Preparation Time: 10 minutes | Cooking Time: 0 minutes (chilling time: 1 hour) | Portion Size: 12 bars

Ingredients:
- 1 cup rolled oats
- 1/2 cup shredded unsweetened coconut
- 1/2 cup sunflower seeds
- 1/4 cup ground flax seeds
- 1/4 cup honey or maple syrup
- 1/4 cup almond butter
- 1 tbsp coconut oil, melted
- 1/2 tsp vanilla extract
- A pinch of salt

Instructions:

In a large mixing bowl, combine the oats, shredded coconut, sunflower seeds, and ground flax seeds. In a small saucepan over low heat, stir together the honey or maple syrup, almond butter, melted coconut oil, vanilla extract, and salt until smooth and well combined. Pour the wet mixture over the dry ingredients and stir until everything is evenly coated. Press the mixture firmly into an 8x8-inch baking dish lined with parchment paper. Refrigerate for at least 1 hour until firm.
Once set, cut into 12 bars and store in an airtight container in the refrigerator.

Nutritional Data:
Calories: 190 | Total Fat: 12g | Saturated Fat: 4g | Cholesterol: 0mg | Sodium: 40mg | Total Carbohydrates: 18g | Dietary Fiber: 4g | Sugars: 7g | Protein: 5g

Lemon-Mint Yogurt Pops

Preparation time: 15 minutes (But 4-6 hours freezing time) | Portion size: Makes 8 pops

Ingredients:
- 2 cups low-fat or non-fat plain yogurt
- 3 tbsp honey or maple syrup (adjust based on desired sweetness)
- Zest and juice of 2 large lemons
- 1/4 cup fresh mint leaves, finely chopped
- 1 tsp vanilla extract
- Popsicle molds or small paper cups and popsicle sticks

Instructions:

In a mixing bowl, whisk together the yogurt, honey or maple syrup, lemon zest, lemon juice, and vanilla extract until smooth and well combined.
Gently fold in the finely chopped mint leaves.
Pour the mixture into the popsicle molds or paper cups, leaving a little space at the top for expansion as they freeze.
If using paper cups, cover each cup with aluminum foil and insert a popsicle stick through the center of the foil (this will help keep the stick upright as it freezes).
Place the popsicle molds or cups in the freezer and allow them to set for at least 4-6 hours, or overnight for best results.
Once frozen, remove the yogurt pops from the molds or paper cups by briefly running them under warm water to loosen.
Serving Suggestion: These soothing yogurt pops are perfect for a summer evening treat or anytime you need a cooling snack.

Nutritional Data: Calories: 70 per pop | Total Fat: 0.5g | Saturated Fat: 0g | Trans Fat: 0g | Cholesterol: 2mg | Sodium: 25mg | Total Carbohydrates: 12g | Dietary Fiber: 0g | Sugars: 11g | Protein: 4g

Carrot and Oat Muffins

Preparation Time: 15 minutes | Cooking Time: 25 minutes | Portion Size: 12 muffins

Ingredients:
- 1 cup whole wheat flour
- 1 cup rolled oats
- 1 tsp baking powder
- 1/2 tsp baking soda
- 1/2 tsp ground cinnamon
- 1/4 tsp ground nutmeg
- 1/4 tsp salt
- 2 large eggs
- 1/2 cup unsweetened applesauce
- 1/4 cup honey or maple syrup
- 1/4 cup olive oil
- 1 tsp vanilla extract
- 1 1/2 cups grated carrots
- 1/4 cup chopped walnuts (optional)

Instructions:

Preheat the oven to 350°F (175°C) and line a muffin tin with paper liners. In a large bowl, mix together the whole wheat flour, rolled oats, baking powder, baking soda, cinnamon, nutmeg, and salt. In a separate bowl, whisk together the eggs, applesauce, honey or maple syrup, olive oil, and vanilla extract. Add the wet ingredients to the dry ingredients and mix until just combined. Fold in the grated carrots and chopped walnuts (if using). Divide the batter evenly among the muffin cups. Bake for 20-25 minutes or until a toothpick inserted into the center of a muffin comes out clean.

Nutritional Data:

Calories: 150 | Total Fat: 7g | Saturated Fat: 1g | Cholesterol: 30mg | Sodium: 120mg | Total Carbohydrates: 20g | Dietary Fiber: 3g | Sugars: 8g | Protein: 3g

Sunflower Seed & Date Balls

Preparation time: 15 minutes (no-bake) | Portion size: Makes 16 balls

Ingredients:
- 1 cup sunflower seeds
- 1 1/2 cups pitted dates
- 1/4 cup shredded unsweetened coconut
- 1 tbsp chia seeds
- 2 tbsp coconut oil, melted
- 1 tsp vanilla extract
- A pinch of salt

Instructions:

Place the sunflower seeds in a food processor and process until they become a fine meal.

Add the pitted dates, shredded coconut, chia seeds, melted coconut oil, vanilla extract, and a pinch of salt to the food processor.

Blend the mixture until it comes together into a sticky dough.

Scoop out tablespoon-sized portions of the mixture and roll them into balls using your hands.

Place the balls on a tray lined with parchment paper.

Refrigerate for at least 1 hour to allow the balls to firm up.

Store in an airtight container in the refrigerator for up to a week.

Serving Suggestion: Perfect for a quick snack, post-workout energy boost, or as a sweet treat after a meal.

Nutritional Data: Calories: 90 per ball | Total Fat: 5g | Saturated Fat: 2g | Trans Fat: 0g | Cholesterol: 0mg | Sodium: 5mg | Total Carbohydrates: 10g | Dietary Fiber: 2g | Sugars: 7g | Protein: 2g

Toasted Almond & Raisin Mix

Preparation time: 5 minutes | Cooking time: 10 minutes | Portion size: Serves 8

Ingredients:
- 1 1/2 cups raw almonds
- 1 cup raisins
- 1 tbsp coconut oil
- 1/2 tsp cinnamon powder
- A pinch of sea salt
- Optional: 1/4 tsp nutmeg for added flavor

Instructions:

Preheat the oven to 350°F (175°C) and line a baking sheet with parchment paper. In a mixing bowl, toss the raw almonds with coconut oil, ensuring they are evenly coated. Spread the almonds on the prepared baking sheet in a single layer. Sprinkle the almonds with cinnamon powder, nutmeg (if using), and a pinch of sea salt. Toast the almonds in the preheated oven for 10 minutes, stirring once or twice to ensure even toasting. Be careful not to burn them. Once toasted, remove from the oven and let them cool. Once cooled, combine the toasted almonds with raisins in a mixing bowl. Mix well. Store in an airtight container at room temperature for up to two weeks.

Serving Suggestion: Enjoy as a nutritious midday snack or sprinkle over salads and yogurts for added crunch and sweetness.

Nutritional Data: Calories: 180 per serving | Total Fat: 12g | Saturated Fat: 2g | Trans Fat: 0g | Cholesterol: 0mg | Sodium: 20mg | Total Carbohydrates: 16g | Dietary Fiber: 4g | Sugars: 9g | Protein: 5g

Honeydew & Cottage Cheese Cup

Preparation time: 10 minutes | Portion size: Serves 4

Ingredients:
- 2 cups honeydew melon, cubed
- 1 1/2 cups low-fat cottage cheese
- 1 tbsp honey (optional, for added sweetness)
- 1 tsp fresh mint, finely chopped
- 1 tbsp chia seeds (for garnish and added nutrition)
- A pinch of sea salt

Instructions:

In a bowl, gently mix the cubed honeydew melon with the finely chopped mint. If you're using honey, drizzle it over the honeydew cubes and give it another gentle stir. In serving cups or bowls, place an equal amount of the cottage cheese at the bottom. Top the cottage cheese with the honeydew-mint mixture. Sprinkle with a pinch of sea salt and garnish with chia seeds on top. Serve immediately and enjoy!

Serving Suggestion: This dish can be consumed as a light breakfast, a healthy snack, or a refreshing dessert.

Nutritional Data: Calories: 115 per serving | Total Fat: 2g | Saturated Fat: 1g | Trans Fat: 0g | Cholesterol: 5mg | Sodium: 240mg | Total Carbohydrates: 15g | Dietary Fiber: 1g | Sugars: 12g | Protein: 10g

Edamame & Sea Salt

Preparation time: 5 minutes | Cooking time: 5 minutes | Portion size: Serves 4

Ingredients:
- 2 cups frozen edamame, shelled
- 1-2 tsp fine sea salt (adjust to taste)
- 1 liter water for boiling

Instructions:

In a medium-sized pot, bring water to a boil. Once boiling, add the frozen edamame to the pot. Cook for 4-5 minutes or until the edamame beans are tender and heated through. Drain the edamame in a colander and place them in a serving bowl. While still warm, sprinkle the edamame with sea salt, tossing them gently to ensure they are evenly coated. Serve immediately as a nutritious snack or side dish.

Serving Suggestion: These are perfect as a healthy snack on their own or can be added to salads for some added protein and crunch.

Nutritional Data: Calories: 95 per serving | Total Fat: 4g | Saturated Fat: 0.5g | Trans Fat: 0g | Cholesterol: 0mg | Sodium: 580mg (based on 1 tsp of sea salt) | Total Carbohydrates: 7g | Dietary Fiber: 3g | Sugars: 2g | Protein: 9g

Rice Pudding with Blueberries

Preparation time: 10 minutes | Cooking time: 25 minutes | Portion size: Serves 6

Ingredients:

- 1 cup Arborio rice or short-grain rice
- 4 cups whole milk (or almond milk for a dairy-free option)
- 1/4 cup granulated sugar or maple syrup
- 1 tsp vanilla extract
- 1/4 tsp salt
- 1 cup fresh blueberries
- Zest of 1 lemon (optional, for added flavor)
- A pinch of ground cinnamon (optional)

Instructions:

In a medium-sized pot, combine the rice, milk, sugar, vanilla extract, and salt.

Bring the mixture to a gentle simmer over medium heat, stirring occasionally.

Reduce heat to low and let the mixture simmer, continuing to stir occasionally, for about 20-25 minutes, or until the rice is tender and the mixture has thickened.

Once cooked, remove the rice pudding from heat and allow it to cool slightly. It will continue to thicken as it cools.

Stir in the fresh blueberries and lemon zest (if using).

Serve warm in individual bowls. If desired, sprinkle with a pinch of ground cinnamon before serving.

Note: This pudding can also be enjoyed cold. If refrigerating, cover the top of the pudding with plastic wrap to prevent a skin from forming.

Nutritional Data: Calories: 210 per serving | Total Fat: 3g | Saturated Fat: 1.5g | Trans Fat: 0g | Cholesterol: 10mg | Sodium: 115mg | Total Carbohydrates: 40g | Dietary Fiber: 1g | Sugars: 18g | Protein: 6g

Green Tea & Lemon Cookies

Preparation time: 15 minutes | Cooking time: 12 minutes | Portion size: Makes 24 cookies

Ingredients:

- 1 cup all-purpose flour
- 1/2 cup almond flour
- 1/2 teaspoon baking powder
- 1/4 teaspoon salt
- 1 tablespoon green tea powder (matcha)
- 1/2 cup unsalted butter, softened
- 1/2 cup granulated sugar
- 1 large egg
- Zest of 1 lemon
- 1 tablespoon freshly squeezed lemon juice

Instructions:

Preheat the oven to 350°F (175°C) and line a baking sheet with parchment paper or a silicone baking mat.

In a medium-sized bowl, whisk together the all-purpose flour, almond flour, baking powder, salt, and green tea powder. Set aside.

In a separate larger bowl, beat the softened butter and sugar together until creamy and smooth. This should take about 2-3 minutes.

Add the egg, lemon zest, and lemon juice to the butter mixture. Mix until combined.

Gradually add the dry ingredients to the wet ingredients, mixing just until incorporated.

Drop rounded tablespoons of dough onto the prepared baking sheet, spacing them about 2 inches apart.

Gently flatten each cookie using the back of a spoon or your fingers.

Bake in the preheated oven for 10-12 minutes or until the edges of the cookies are lightly golden.

Allow the cookies to cool on the baking sheet for a few minutes before transferring them to a wire rack to cool completely.

Nutritional Data: Calories: 80 per cookie | Total Fat: 4.5g | Saturated Fat: 2.5g | Trans Fat: 0g | Cholesterol: 15mg | Sodium: 25mg | Total Carbohydrates: 9g | Dietary Fiber: 0.5g | Sugars: 4g | Protein: 1.5g

Banana & Almond Butter Slices

Preparation time: 10 minutes   (Chill time: 1 hour) | Portion size: Makes 12 slices

Ingredients:

- 3 ripe bananas
- 1/2 cup almond butter, smooth or crunchy based on preference
- 2 tablespoons honey or maple syrup (optional for added sweetness)
- 1 teaspoon vanilla extract
- A pinch of salt
- 1/4 cup chopped almonds for garnish
- 1 tablespoon chia seeds (optional for added texture)

Instructions:

Peel and slice the bananas into 1/2-inch thick rounds. In a medium-sized bowl, combine the almond butter, honey (or maple syrup if using), vanilla extract, and a pinch of salt. Mix until smooth. Lay the banana slices flat on a plate or tray. Spread a generous amount of the almond butter mixture onto half of the banana slices. Top with the remaining banana slices, pressing down gently to form a sandwich. Sprinkle the tops with chopped almonds and chia seeds, if using. Place the banana and almond butter slices in the freezer for at least 1 hour, or until they are firm. Once chilled, they're ready to be served! Enjoy immediately or store in an airtight container in the freezer for up to a week.

Note: These slices are best enjoyed chilled. If left out for an extended period, they can become soft and messy.

Nutritional Data: Calories: 105 per slice | Total Fat: 6g | Saturated Fat: 0.5g | Trans Fat: 0g | Cholesterol: 0mg | Sodium: 2mg | Total Carbohydrates: 12g | Dietary Fiber: 2g | Sugars: 7g | Protein: 2.5g

Seed Crackers with Avocado Dip

Preparation time: 20 minutes | Cooking time: 50 minutes | Portion size: Serves 6

Ingredients for the Seed Crackers:
- 1/2 cup flax seeds
- 1/4 cup chia seeds
- 1/4 cup pumpkin seeds (pepitas)
- 1/4 cup sunflower seeds
- 1/4 teaspoon salt
- 1 cup water

Ingredients for the Avocado Dip:
- 2 ripe avocados
- Juice of 1 lemon
- 1 clove garlic, minced (optional)
- Salt to taste
- 1 tablespoon olive oil
- 1 tablespoon chopped fresh cilantro (optional)

Instructions:

For the Seed Crackers:
Preheat the oven to 300°F (150°C).

In a large mixing bowl, combine flax seeds, chia seeds, pumpkin seeds, sunflower seeds, and salt.

Add water and mix well. Let the mixture sit for 15-20 minutes, or until the water is absorbed and a thick, gel-like consistency forms.

Spread the mixture thinly and evenly on a parchment-lined baking sheet.

Bake for about 50 minutes, checking occasionally. Once the crackers are crispy and golden, remove them from the oven and let them cool completely.

Break into desired cracker sizes.

For the Avocado Dip:
Cut the avocados in half, remove the pits, and scoop the flesh into a bowl.

Add the lemon juice, garlic (if using), salt, and olive oil.

Mash the ingredients together until smooth. Adjust seasoning if necessary.

Stir in the chopped cilantro, if using.

Serve the seed crackers with the fresh avocado dip. Enjoy!

Nutritional Data: Calories: 230 per serving | Total Fat: 18g | Saturated Fat: 2.5g | Trans Fat: 0g | Cholesterol: 0mg | Sodium: 105mg | Total Carbohydrates: 15g | Dietary Fiber: 9g | Sugars: 1g | Protein: 6g

Date & Walnut Energy Bites

Preparation time: 15 minutes   (No cook, just chill) | Portion size: Makes 12 bites

Ingredients:

- 1 cup pitted Medjool dates
- 1 cup walnuts
- 1/2 teaspoon vanilla extract
- Pinch of salt
- 2 tablespoons shredded coconut (optional for coating)

Instructions:

In a food processor, combine the pitted dates, walnuts, vanilla extract, and a pinch of salt. Blend until the mixture forms a sticky dough-like consistency.

Using clean hands, take about a tablespoon of the mixture and roll it into a ball. Repeat with the remaining mixture until all of it has been used.

If using, spread the shredded coconut on a plate. Roll the energy bites in the coconut, ensuring they are well coated.

Place the energy bites on a tray or plate lined with parchment paper. Refrigerate for at least an hour to set.

Once set, transfer the energy bites to an airtight container and store in the refrigerator. They're best enjoyed cold!

Nutritional Data: Calories: 95 per bite | Total Fat: 5g | Saturated Fat: 0.5g | Trans Fat: 0g | Cholesterol: 0mg | Sodium: 2mg | Total Carbohydrates: 12g | Dietary Fiber: 2g | Sugars: 9g | Protein: 2g

Chapter 8: Drinks

The significance of a beverage goes far beyond its ability to simply quench one's thirst. It possesses the remarkable power to uplift spirits, provide solace to the soul, and offer nourishment to the body. Yet, for individuals who are diligently managing acid reflux, the choice of beverages isn't always a simple matter. That beloved cup of aromatic coffee, the zesty citrus juice, or the fizzy soda can sometimes become sources of discomfort that linger for hours.

However, there's no need to fret, for within the pages of this chapter dedicated to "Drinks Recipes," we present a curated collection of beverages designed with the specific needs of those seeking relief from acid reflux in mind. From the warm, comforting brews that cocoon your senses to the cool, revitalizing concoctions that refresh your palate, each recipe has been meticulously crafted to ensure that it not only tantalizes your taste buds but also treats your digestive system with care and consideration.

With these beverage recipes at your disposal, you can now relish a cup of goodness that not only satisfies your cravings but also prioritizes your comfort. So, dive into this chapter with the understanding that your beverage can be a source of pleasure, nourishment, and, above all, relief from acid reflux-related discomfort.

Recipes

Green Ginger Tea

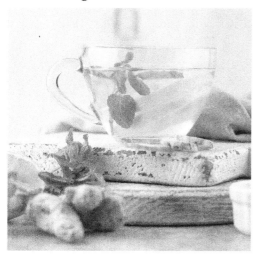

Preparation time: 5 minutes | Cooking time: 10 minutes | Portion size: Serves 2

Ingredients:

- 2 cups of water
- 1 green tea bag or 1 tablespoon loose green tea leaves
- 1-inch piece of fresh ginger, thinly sliced
- 1 teaspoon honey or to taste (optional)
- A slice of lemon (optional)

Instructions:

In a pot, bring the water to a boil. Once boiling, reduce to a simmer.

Add the ginger slices to the simmering water. Let them infuse for about 7 minutes.

Turn off the heat and add the green tea. Allow it to steep for 2-3 minutes. If you're using loose leaves, you might want to strain the tea.

Remove the tea bag or strain the tea to remove the leaves and ginger slices.

Pour the tea into cups. If desired, add honey for a touch of sweetness and a slice of lemon for a hint of citrus.

Enjoy your soothing tea while warm!

Nutritional Data: Calories: 5 (without honey) | Total Fat: 0g | Saturated Fat: 0g | Trans Fat: 0g | Cholesterol: 0mg | Sodium: 9mg | Total Carbohydrates: 1g | Dietary Fiber: 0g | Sugars: 0g (1g with honey) | Protein: 0g

Note: Nutritional data can vary based on the specific brands and amounts of ingredients used. It's always a good idea to double-check with a nutrition calculator if exact accuracy is essential.

Chamomile & Lavender Infusion

Preparation time: 3 minutes | Cooking time: 10 minutes | Portion size: Serves 2

Ingredients:
- 2 cups of water
- 2 chamomile tea bags or 2 tablespoons loose chamomile flowers
- 1 teaspoon dried lavender buds
- Honey or stevia to taste (optional)
- A slice of lemon (optional)

Instructions:

In a kettle or pot, bring the water to a boil. Once boiling, remove from heat.

Add the chamomile tea bags or loose flowers and the dried lavender buds to the hot water.

Allow the mixture to steep for about 8-10 minutes.

Remove the tea bags or strain the infusion to remove the loose flowers and lavender buds.

Pour the infusion into cups. Add honey or stevia for sweetness if desired, and a slice of lemon for a subtle citrus touch.

Relax and enjoy the calming effects of this infusion.

Nutritional Data: Calories: 2 (without honey) | Total Fat: 0g | Saturated Fat: 0g | Trans Fat: 0g | Cholesterol: 0mg | Sodium: 8mg | Total Carbohydrates: 0.5g | Dietary Fiber: 0g | Sugars: 0g (variable with honey or stevia) | Protein: 0g

Berry & Banana Blend

Preparation time: 5 minutes | Portion size: Serves 2

Ingredients:
- 1 ripe banana, peeled and sliced
- 1 cup mixed berries (like strawberries, blueberries, and raspberries)
- 1 cup almond milk (unsweetened)
- 1 tablespoon chia seeds (optional for added nutrition)
- 1 teaspoon honey or stevia (optional for sweetness)
- A handful of ice cubes

Instructions:

Place the sliced banana, mixed berries, almond milk, and chia seeds (if using) into a blender.

If you desire a sweeter taste, add honey or stevia.

Add the ice cubes last.

Blend until smooth and creamy.

Pour into glasses and enjoy immediately for a refreshing treat.

Nutritional Data: Calories: 145 | Total Fat: 3g | Saturated Fat: 0.2g | Trans Fat: 0g | Cholesterol: 0mg | Sodium: 80mg | Total Carbohydrates: 29g | Dietary Fiber: 6g | Sugars: 17g | Protein: 3g

Papaya Punch

Preparation time: 10 minutes | Portion size: Serves 4

Ingredients:

- 2 cups ripe papaya, peeled, deseeded, and diced
- 1 cup coconut water (unsweetened)
- 1 tablespoon fresh lime juice
- 1 teaspoon honey or stevia (optional for sweetness)
- A few sprigs of fresh mint
- 1 cup sparkling water or club soda (chilled)
- Ice cubes, as required

Instructions:

In a blender, combine the diced papaya, coconut water, lime juice, and honey or stevia if you're adding sweetness. Blend until smooth.

Fill glasses halfway with the papaya mixture.

Top each glass with chilled sparkling water or club soda.

Garnish with a sprig of fresh mint.

Add ice cubes and give a gentle stir.

Serve immediately and enjoy the calming effects of the Peaceful Papaya Punch.

Nutritional Data: Calories: 65 | Total Fat: 0.3g | Saturated Fat: 0.1g | Trans Fat: 0g | Cholesterol: 0mg | Sodium: 40mg | Total Carbohydrates: 16g | Dietary Fiber: 2.5g | Sugars: 12g | Protein: 1g

Carrot & Apple Juice Blend

Preparation time: 15 minutes | Portion size: Serves 4

Ingredients:

- 4 large carrots, washed and peeled
- 2 medium-sized apples, washed and cored
- 1-inch piece of fresh ginger, peeled
- 1 tablespoon fresh lemon juice
- 1 cup of water
- Ice cubes, as required

Instructions:

Cut the carrots and apples into small chunks that will easily fit into your juicer.

Pass the carrots, apples, and ginger through the juicer.

Collect the juice in a large pitcher.

Add the fresh lemon juice and water to the pitcher and stir well.

Refrigerate for about 30 minutes or until chilled.

Pour the juice into glasses, add ice cubes if desired, and serve immediately.

Nutritional Data: Calories: 95 | Total Fat: 0.4g | Saturated Fat: 0.1g | Trans Fat: 0g | Cholesterol: 0mg | Sodium: 65mg | Total Carbohydrates: 24g | Dietary Fiber: 5g | Sugars: 18g | Protein: 1.2g

Watermelon Hydration

Preparation time: 10 minutes | Portion size: Serves 4

Ingredients:
- 4 cups of seedless watermelon, cubed
- 1 cup of fresh coconut water
- 1 tablespoon of fresh mint leaves, finely chopped
- Juice of 1 lime
- Ice cubes, as required

Instructions:

In a blender, combine the watermelon cubes and coconut water. Blend until smooth.

Strain the mixture through a fine sieve to remove any pulp, if desired.

Add the lime juice and finely chopped mint to the strained juice. Stir well.

Refrigerate for about 20-30 minutes or until chilled.

Serve the hydration in glasses with ice cubes.

Note: This refreshing drink is perfect for summer days and provides hydration with the added benefits of watermelon and coconut water.

Nutritional Data: Calories: 60 | Total Fat: 0.2g | Saturated Fat: 0.1g | Trans Fat: 0g | Cholesterol: 0mg | Sodium: 40mg | Total Carbohydrates: 15g | Dietary Fiber: 0.5g | Sugars: 12g | Protein: 1g

Dandelion Root Tea

Preparation time: 5 minutes | Cooking time: 10 minutes | Portion size: Serves 2

Ingredients:
- 2 tablespoons of dried dandelion root
- 4 cups of water
- Optional: 1 teaspoon of honey or a slice of lemon for flavor

Instructions:

In a saucepan, bring the water to a boil.

Once boiling, add the dried dandelion root.

Reduce the heat and let it simmer for about 7-10 minutes.

Remove from heat and strain the tea to remove the dandelion root.

Pour the tea into cups and, if desired, add honey or a slice of lemon for flavor.

Note: Dandelion root tea is known for its potential liver-detoxifying properties and can be a gentle beverage choice for those with acid reflux.

Nutritional Data: Calories: 5 | Total Fat: 0g | Saturated Fat: 0g | Trans Fat: 0g | Cholesterol: 0mg | Sodium: 12mg | Total Carbohydrates: 1g | Dietary Fiber: 0g | Sugars: 0g | Protein: 0g

Turmeric & Almond Milk Latte

Preparation time: 5 minutes | Cooking time: 5 minutes | Portion size: Serves 2

Ingredients:

- 2 cups unsweetened almond milk
- 1 teaspoon ground turmeric
- 1/4 teaspoon ground cinnamon
- A pinch of black pepper (to enhance the absorption of turmeric)
- Optional: 1 teaspoon of honey or maple syrup for sweetness
- Optional: 1/4 teaspoon of ground ginger for added warmth

Instructions:

In a saucepan, gently heat the almond milk on medium heat, but do not let it boil.

As the milk is heating, add the turmeric, cinnamon, and black pepper. If using, also add the ground ginger.

Whisk continuously to ensure the spices are well incorporated and to prevent the milk from forming a skin.

Once hot, remove from heat. If desired, sweeten with honey or maple syrup to your preference.

Pour into mugs and serve immediately. A sprinkle of cinnamon on top can be a lovely touch.

Note: Turmeric contains curcumin, an anti-inflammatory compound, which can be soothing for the stomach and digestion.

Nutritional Data: Calories: 40 | Total Fat: 3g | Saturated Fat: 0g | Trans Fat: 0g | Cholesterol: 0mg | Sodium: 180mg | Total Carbohydrates: 2g | Dietary Fiber: 0.5g | Sugars: 1g (if no sweetener added) | Protein: 1g

Zesty Lemon & Cucumber Cooler

Preparation time: 10 minutes | Portion size: Serves 4

Ingredients:

- 1 large cucumber, thinly sliced
- 2 lemons, juiced
- 4 cups of cold water
- 1 tablespoon of honey or maple syrup (optional)
- A handful of fresh mint leaves
- Ice cubes, for serving

Instructions:

In a large pitcher, combine the sliced cucumber, lemon juice, and cold water.

If a touch of sweetness is desired, add honey or maple syrup and stir well until dissolved.

Add fresh mint leaves, lightly bruised to release their flavor.

Chill in the refrigerator for at least 1 hour to allow the flavors to meld.

Serve over ice cubes in glasses.

Note: This refreshing cooler is not only hydrating but also beneficial for the stomach, thanks to the soothing properties of cucumber and mint.

Nutritional Data: Calories: 25 | Total Fat: 0g | Saturated Fat: 0g | Trans Fat: 0g | Cholesterol: 0mg | Sodium: 10mg | Total Carbohydrates: 7g | Dietary Fiber: 1g | Sugars: 4g (if sweetened with honey) | Protein: 0.5g

Strawberry & Oat Smoothie

Preparation time: 5 minutes | Portion size: Serves 2

Ingredients:
- 1 cup fresh or frozen strawberries
- 1/2 cup rolled oats
- 1 cup almond milk (unsweetened)
- 1 ripe banana
- 1 tablespoon chia seeds
- 1 teaspoon honey or maple syrup (optional)
- A few ice cubes (if using fresh strawberries)

Instructions:

In a blender, combine strawberries, rolled oats, almond milk, banana, and chia seeds. Blend on high until smooth. If you prefer a sweeter taste, add honey or maple syrup and blend again to mix well. If using fresh strawberries, add ice cubes and blend until the smoothie reaches your desired consistency. Pour into glasses and serve immediately.

Note: The combination of oats and chia seeds in this smoothie provides a gentle, soothing texture that can be beneficial for those with acid reflux. Opting for almond milk instead of dairy milk further makes this recipe reflux-friendly.

Nutritional Data: Calories: 210 | Total Fat: 4.5g | Saturated Fat: 0.5g | Trans Fat: 0g | Cholesterol: 0mg | Sodium: 80mg | Total Carbohydrates: 40g | Dietary Fiber: 7g | Sugars: 14g | Protein: 5g

Peach & Ginger Iced Tea

Preparation time: 10 minutes | Cooking time: 15 minutes | Portion size: Serves 4

Ingredients:
- 4 cups water
- 2 fresh peaches, pitted and sliced
- 2-inch piece of fresh ginger, thinly sliced
- 2 tea bags of your choice (green or herbal tea recommended for acid reflux sufferers)
- 1 tablespoon honey or maple syrup (optional)
- Ice cubes
- Fresh mint leaves for garnish (optional)

Instructions:

In a saucepan, bring water to a boil. Add the sliced peaches and ginger to the boiling water. Reduce heat and let simmer for 10 minutes. Remove from heat and add the tea bags. Allow to steep for 5 minutes. Discard the tea bags, then strain the tea to remove the peaches and ginger. If desired, some peach slices can be reserved for garnish. Let the tea cool to room temperature. Once cooled, refrigerate until chilled. If you prefer a sweeter taste, stir in honey or maple syrup until dissolved. Serve over ice cubes and garnish with reserved peach slices or fresh mint leaves if desired.

Note: Ginger is known for its soothing properties and can be beneficial for those with acid reflux, while peach adds a natural sweetness and refreshing flavor to the tea.

Nutritional Data: Calories: 30 | Total Fat: 0g | Saturated Fat: 0g | Trans Fat: 0g | Cholesterol: 0mg | Sodium: 10mg | Total Carbohydrates: 8g | Dietary Fiber: 1g | Sugars: 6g | Protein: 0.5g

Blueberry Basil Lemonade

Preparation time: 15 minutes | Cooking time: 5 minutes | Portion size: Serves 4

Ingredients:
- 1 cup fresh blueberries
- 1/2 cup fresh basil leaves, plus more for garnish
- 1/2 cup freshly squeezed lemon juice (about 3-4 lemons)
- 1/4 cup honey or maple syrup (or adjust to taste)
- 4 cups water
- Ice cubes
- Lemon slices for garnish (optional)

Instructions:

In a saucepan, combine blueberries, basil leaves, and 1 cup of water. Bring to a gentle boil, then reduce heat and simmer for about 5 minutes until the blueberries have released their juices. Strain the blueberry-basil mixture, discarding the solids. Allow the liquid to cool to room temperature. In a large pitcher, combine the blueberry-basil liquid, fresh lemon juice, honey or maple syrup, and the remaining 3 cups of water. Stir well until everything is well-mixed. Taste and adjust sweetness as needed. Serve the lemonade over ice cubes, garnished with additional basil leaves and lemon slices if desired.

Note: Basil adds an aromatic twist to this refreshing lemonade, while blueberries provide a delightful natural sweetness and vibrant color.

Nutritional Data: Calories: 70 | Total Fat: 0.2g | Saturated Fat: 0g | Trans Fat: 0g | Cholesterol: 0mg | Sodium: 12mg | Total Carbohydrates: 18g | Dietary Fiber: 1g | Sugars: 15g | Protein: 0.5g

Herbal Infusion with Rose Hips

Preparation time: 5 minutes | Cooking time: 10 minutes | Portion size: Serves 4

Ingredients:
- 4 cups of water
- 2 tablespoons dried rose hips
- 1 tablespoon chamomile flowers
- 1 tablespoon peppermint leaves
- 1 tablespoon honey or maple syrup (optional for sweetness)
- Lemon slices for garnish (optional)

Instructions:

Bring the water to a boil in a kettle or a saucepan. In a teapot or heatproof container, combine the dried rose hips, chamomile flowers, and peppermint leaves. Pour the boiling water over the herbs and let the mixture steep for about 8-10 minutes. Strain the infusion, discarding the solids. If desired, sweeten with honey or maple syrup to taste. Pour into cups and garnish with a slice of lemon if using.

Note: Rose hips provide a delightful tanginess while the chamomile and peppermint provide calming properties to this infusion. Perfect for sipping before bedtime or any time you wish to relax.

Nutritional Data: Calories: 10 (without honey or syrup) | Total Fat: 0g | Saturated Fat: 0g | Trans Fat: 0g | Cholesterol: 0mg | Sodium: 8mg | Total Carbohydrates: 2.5g (without honey or syrup) | Dietary Fiber: 0.8g | Sugars: 0g (without honey or syrup) | Protein: 0.1g

Rooibos & Vanilla Steamer

Preparation time: 5 minutes | Cooking time: 10 minutes | Portion size: Serves 4

Ingredients:
- 4 cups of water
- 4 rooibos tea bags or 4 tablespoons loose rooibos tea
- 1 cup unsweetened almond milk (or any non-dairy milk of your choice)
- 2 teaspoons pure vanilla extract
- Honey or maple syrup to taste (optional for sweetness)
- A sprinkle of ground cinnamon for garnish (optional)

Instructions:

Bring the water to a boil in a kettle or a saucepan.

Place the rooibos tea bags or loose tea in a teapot or heatproof container.

Pour the boiling water over the tea and allow to steep for 5-7 minutes.

In a separate saucepan, gently heat the almond milk until it's warm but not boiling.

Remove the tea bags or strain the tea if using loose tea.

Add the vanilla extract to the tea, followed by the warmed almond milk.

Stir gently to combine. If desired, sweeten with honey or maple syrup to taste.

Pour into mugs and sprinkle with a touch of ground cinnamon if using.

Note: Rooibos is naturally caffeine-free and has a mild, slightly sweet taste. Combined with vanilla and almond milk, it creates a comforting beverage perfect for relaxation.

Nutritional Data: Calories: 30 | Total Fat: 1g | Saturated Fat: 0g | Trans Fat: 0g | Cholesterol: 0mg | Sodium: 55mg | Total Carbohydrates: 4g (without honey or syrup) | Dietary Fiber: 0.5g | Sugars: 1g (without honey or syrup) | Protein: 1g

Licorice & Fennel Tea

Preparation time: 5 minutes | Cooking time: 15 minutes | Portion size: Serves 4

Ingredients:

- 1 tablespoon licorice root, dried and chopped
- 1 tablespoon fennel seeds
- 4 cups of water
- Honey or maple syrup to taste (optional for sweetness)
- Fresh mint leaves for garnish (optional)

Instructions:

In a medium-sized saucepan, bring the water to a gentle boil. Add the licorice root and fennel seeds. Reduce the heat, cover, and let simmer for about 10-12 minutes. Remove from heat and strain the tea into cups or a teapot, discarding the licorice and fennel. If desired, sweeten with honey or maple syrup to taste. Garnish with fresh mint leaves if using.

Note: Both licorice and fennel are known for their soothing properties which can be beneficial for those with acid reflux. The sweet flavor of licorice combined with the aromatic essence of fennel creates a gentle and calming tea perfect for bedtime relaxation.

Nutritional Data: Calories: 8 | Total Fat: 0.1g | Saturated Fat: 0g | Trans Fat: 0g | Cholesterol: 0mg | Sodium: 10mg | Total Carbohydrates: 2g (without honey or syrup) | Dietary Fiber: 0.2g | Sugars: 0.5g (without honey or syrup) | Protein: 0.2g

Quencher: Coconut & Pineapple Blend

Preparation time: 10 minutes | Portion size: Serves 4

Ingredients:

- 2 cups fresh pineapple chunks
- 1 can (14 oz.) of coconut milk (full-fat or light, depending on preference)
- 1 cup of coconut water
- 1 tablespoon chia seeds (optional for added fiber and texture)
- Ice cubes (optional for a colder drink)
- A pinch of salt
- Fresh pineapple slices and mint leaves for garnish

Instructions:

In a blender, combine the pineapple chunks, coconut milk, coconut water, chia seeds (if using), and a pinch of salt. Blend on high speed until smooth and creamy.
If desired, add ice cubes and blend again until well-mixed and chilled.
Pour the blend into glasses and garnish with fresh pineapple slices and mint leaves.

Note: Pineapple contains bromelain, an enzyme that helps in digestion, and when combined with the soothing properties of coconut, this blend serves as a gentle drink ideal for those with acid reflux.

Nutritional Data: Calories: 210 | Total Fat: 14g | Saturated Fat: 12g | Trans Fat: 0g | Cholesterol: 0mg | Sodium: 90mg | Total Carbohydrates: 21g | Dietary Fiber: 3g | Sugars: 14g | Protein: 2g

Mango & Aloe Vera Elixir

Preparation time: 10 minutes | Portion size: Serves 4

Ingredients:

- 2 ripe mangoes, peeled and pitted
- 1 cup aloe vera juice (ensure it's food-grade and suitable for consumption)
- 2 cups of filtered water
- 1 tablespoon fresh lemon juice
- 1 tablespoon honey or agave syrup (adjust based on sweetness preference)
- Ice cubes (optional for a colder drink)
- Mint leaves for garnish

Instructions:

In a blender, combine the mango chunks, aloe vera juice, water, lemon juice, and honey or agave syrup. Blend on high speed until smooth and well-mixed. Taste and adjust sweetness, if necessary. If desired, add ice cubes and blend again until chilled. Pour the elixir into glasses and garnish with fresh mint leaves.

Note: Mangoes are rich in vitamins, while aloe vera is known for its soothing properties, making this elixir a gentle and delightful option for those with acid reflux.

Nutritional Data: Calories: 120 | Total Fat: 0.5g | Saturated Fat: 0.1g | Trans Fat: 0g | Cholesterol: 0mg | Sodium: 15mg | Total Carbohydrates: 30g | Dietary Fiber: 2g | Sugars: 27g | Protein: 1g

Tisane with Lemon Balm & Mint

Preparation time: 5 minutes | Cooking time: 10 minutes | Portion size: Serves 4

Ingredients:

- 1/4 cup fresh lemon balm leaves, loosely packed
- 1/4 cup fresh mint leaves, loosely packed
- 4 cups of filtered water
- 1 tablespoon honey or agave syrup (optional, adjust based on sweetness preference)
- Lemon slices for garnish (optional)
- Fresh sprigs of mint for garnish

Instructions:

In a pot, bring the water to a gentle boil. Once boiling, remove from heat and add in the lemon balm and mint leaves. Cover the pot with a lid and allow the herbs to steep for about 8-10 minutes. Strain the tea into cups, discarding the leaves. If desired, sweeten with honey or agave syrup, stirring well. Garnish with a slice of lemon and a sprig of mint.

Note: Lemon balm and mint are both known for their calming properties and ability to support digestion, making this tisane a delightful and beneficial drink for those experiencing acid reflux.

Nutritional Data: Calories: 10 (without added sweetener) | Total Fat: 0g | Saturated Fat: 0g | Trans Fat: 0g | Cholesterol: 0mg | Sodium: 10mg | Total Carbohydrates: 2.5g (with honey or agave) | Dietary Fiber: 0g | Sugars: 2g (with honey or agave) | Protein: 0g

Maple & Pecan Milkshake

Preparation time: 10 minutes | Portion size: Serves 2

Ingredients:

- 2 cups almond milk (or other non-dairy milk of choice)
- 1/4 cup pecans, plus extra for garnish
- 2 tablespoons pure maple syrup
- 1 teaspoon vanilla extract
- A pinch of sea salt
- 1 cup ice cubes
- Whipped coconut cream for topping (optional)

Instructions:

In a blender, combine almond milk, pecans, maple syrup, vanilla extract, and a pinch of sea salt. Blend on high speed until the pecans are finely ground and the mixture is smooth. Add ice cubes and blend again until the shake is chilled and frothy. Pour the milkshake into glasses. If desired, top with a dollop of whipped coconut cream and a sprinkle of chopped pecans.

Nutritional Data: Calories: 180 | Total Fat: 9g | Saturated Fat: 0.8g | Trans Fat: 0g | Cholesterol: 0mg | Sodium: 90mg | Total Carbohydrates: 21g | Dietary Fiber: 2g | Sugars: 16g | Protein: 3g

Slippery Elm Bark Soother

Preparation time: 5 minutes | Cooking time: 10 minutes | Portion size: Serves 1

Ingredients:

- 1 tablespoon slippery elm bark powder
- 2 cups water
- 1 teaspoon raw honey (optional)
- A pinch of cinnamon (optional)

Instructions:

In a saucepan, add the water and slippery elm bark powder.
Stir the mixture continuously over medium heat until it thickens. This usually takes about 10 minutes.
Once thickened, remove from heat and allow to cool slightly.
If desired, stir in raw honey for a touch of sweetness and a sprinkle of cinnamon for added flavor.
Pour into a mug and drink while warm.
Note: Slippery elm bark has been used traditionally for various ailments, including soothing the stomach and alleviating acid reflux symptoms. Its mucilaginous nature coats the esophagus and stomach, providing relief from acid irritation.

Nutritional Data: Calories: 30 (without honey) / 65 (with honey) | Total Fat: 0g | Saturated Fat: 0g | Trans Fat: 0g | Cholesterol: 0mg | Sodium: 10mg | Total Carbohydrates: 8g (without honey) / 18g (with honey) | Dietary Fiber: 2g | Sugars: 0g (without honey) / 8g (with honey) | Protein: 0g

Chapter 9: 60 - Day Meal Plan

Embarking on a journey to manage and alleviate acid reflux doesn't mean you're relegated to bland and uninspiring meals. In fact, the next 60 days will be a culinary adventure, coupling delightful dishes with healing properties. This carefully curated 60-day meal plan is designed not only to minimize triggers of acid reflux but also to provide nutritious, balanced, and delicious meals that can be enjoyed by everyone, not just those suffering from reflux. Each day is structured to give you a mix of proteins, grains, and vegetables, ensuring you get the necessary nutrients while keeping your symptoms at bay. As you navigate this plan, remember that every individual's body is different. You may find that some foods work better for you than others, and that's okay. Use this meal plan as a blueprint, adjusting where necessary based on your personal experiences and preferences.

Day 1
- **Breakfast**: Golden Turmeric Oatmeal
- **Lunch**: Spinach, Quinoa, and Avocado Salad
- **Snack**: Carrot & Cucumber Pinwheels
- **Dinner**: Grilled Tilapia with Herbed Quinoa

Day 2
- **Breakfast**: Soothing Ginger-Pear Smoothie
- **Lunch**: Rice Pilaf with Almonds
- **Snack**: Banana & Almond Butter Slices
- **Dinner**: Herb-Infused Chicken Breast with Steamed Veggies & Pesto

Day 3
- **Breakfast**: Avocado Toast on Sprouted Bread
- **Lunch**: Turmeric Chicken Wraps
- **Snack**: Coconut and Sunflower Seed Energy Bars
- **Dinner**: Eggplant & Chickpea Curry

Day 4
- **Breakfast**: Flaxseed Morning Muffins
- **Lunch**: Silky Sesame & Chicken Cold Noodles
- **Snack**: Sunflower Seed & Date Balls
- **Dinner**: Butternut & Barley Risotto

Day 5
- **Breakfast**: Quinoa Porridge
- **Lunch**: Broccoli & Quinoa Bowl
- **Snack**: Honeydew & Cottage Cheese Cup
- **Dinner**: Spaghetti Squash with Olive Tapenade

Day 6
- **Breakfast**: Coconut & Blueberry Chia Pudding
- **Lunch**: Cannellini Bean and Carrot Soup
- **Snack**: Seed Crackers with Avocado Dip
- **Dinner**: Lemon-Poached Cod with Spinach

Day 7
- **Breakfast**: Banana & Almond Butter Oats
- **Lunch**: Polenta with Sautéed Greens
- **Snack**: Date & Walnut Energy Bites
- **Dinner**: Quinoa and Roasted Root Vegetable Salad

Day 8
- **Breakfast**: Whole Grain Pancakes with a side of Mint & Melon Medley
- **Lunch**: Zucchini Noodles with Pesto
- **Snack**: Dill & Carrot Hummus with Wheat Crackers
- **Dinner**: Mushroom & Brown Rice Bowl

Day 9
- **Breakfast**: Buckwheat & Berry Bowl
- **Lunch**: Steamed Sea Bass Fillet with Fennel
- **Snack**: Green Tea & Lemon Cookies
- **Dinner**: Fennel & White Bean Stew

Day 10
- **Breakfast**: Refined-Sugar-Free Apple & Cinnamon Crepes
- **Lunch**: Hummus & Pita with a side of Roasted Vegetable Platter
- **Snack**: Mango Rice Cakes
- **Dinner**: Baked Quinoa and Spinach Patties

Day 11
- **Breakfast**: Cinnamon Rice Cereal Delight
- **Lunch**: Tuna & Avocado Salad
- **Snack**: Toasted Almond & Raisin Mix
- **Dinner**: Tofu Stir-Fry with Veggies

Day 12
- **Breakfast**: Omega-Rich Chia & Hemp Seed Parfait
- **Lunch**: Pea & Mint Risotto
- **Snack**: Lemon-Mint Yogurt Pops
- **Dinner**: Savory Stuffed Acorn Squash

Day 13
- **Breakfast**: Oatmeal with Apple and Chia Seeds
- **Lunch**: Rustic Root Vegetable Medley
- **Snack**: Edamame & Sea Salt
- **Dinner**: Quiche with Spinach & Feta

Day 14
- **Breakfast**: Tofu & Spinach Breakfast Scramble
- **Lunch**: Golden Beet & Barley Bowl with Lemon Zest
- **Snack**: Rice Pudding with Blueberries
- **Dinner**: Chickpea and Sweet Potato Patties

Day 15
- **Breakfast**: Greens Morning Juice with a side of Whole Grain Pancakes
- **Lunch**: Spinach, Quinoa, and Avocado Salad with a side of Roasted Vegetable Platter
- **Snack**: Toasted Oats & Banana Bars
- **Dinner**: Baked Falafel with Tzatziki

Day 16
- **Breakfast**: Banana & Almond Butter Oats
- **Lunch**: Soothing Spinach & Tofu Curry
- **Snack**: Date & Walnut Energy Bites
- **Dinner**: Steamed Veggies & Pesto with Lettuce Wrap with Chicken and Avocado

Day 17
- **Breakfast**: Avocado Toast on Sprouted Bread
- **Lunch**: Eggplant & Chickpea Curry
- **Snack**: Coconut and Sunflower Seed Energy Bars
- **Dinner**: Lemon-Poached Cod with Spinach

Day 18
- **Breakfast**: Coconut & Blueberry Chia Pudding
- **Lunch**: Turmeric Chicken Wraps with a side of Golden Beet & Barley Bowl with Lemon Zest
- **Snack**: Carrot & Cucumber Pinwheels
- **Dinner**: Butternut & Barley Risotto

Day 19
- **Breakfast**: Flaxseed Morning Muffins
- **Lunch**: Polenta with Sautéed Greens
- **Snack**: Honeydew & Cottage Cheese Cup
- **Dinner**: Fennel & White Bean Stew

Day 20
- **Breakfast**: Cinnamon Rice Cereal Delight
- **Lunch**: Tuna & Avocado Salad with a side of Broccoli & Quinoa Bowl
- **Snack**: Green Tea & Lemon Cookies
- **Dinner**: Spaghetti Squash with Olive Tapenade

Day 21
- **Breakfast**: Soothing Ginger-Pear Smoothie with a side of Refined-Sugar-Free Apple & Cinnamon Crepes
- **Lunch**: Cannellini Bean and Carrot Soup
- **Snack**: Dill & Carrot Hummus with Carrot Sticks
- **Dinner**: Quiche with Spinach & Feta

Day 22
- **Breakfast**: Golden Turmeric Oatmeal with a side of Mint & Melon Medley
- **Lunch**: Broccoli & Quinoa Bowl with a side of Silky Sesame & Chicken Cold Noodles
- **Snack**: Lemon-Mint Yogurt Pops
- **Dinner**: Mushroom & Brown Rice Bowl

Day 23
- **Breakfast**: Quinoa Porridge with a side of Avocado Toast on Sprouted Bread
- **Lunch**: Spinach, Quinoa, and Avocado Salad with a side of Pea & Mint Risotto
- **Snack**: Mango Rice Cakes
- **Dinner**: Baked Quinoa and Spinach Patties

Day 24
- **Breakfast**: Banana & Almond Butter Oats
- **Lunch**: Golden Beet & Barley Bowl with Lemon Zest with a side of Hummus & Pita
- **Snack**: Date & Walnut Energy Bites
- **Dinner**: Fennel & White Bean Stew

Day 25
- **Breakfast**: Omega-Rich Chia & Hemp Seed Parfait
- **Lunch**: Polenta with Sautéed Greens with a side of Roasted Vegetable Platter
- **Snack**: Coconut and Sunflower Seed Energy Bars
- **Dinner**: Savory Stuffed Acorn Squash

Day 26
- **Breakfast**: Flaxseed Morning Muffins with a side of Soothing Ginger-Pear Smoothie
- **Lunch**: Silky Sesame & Chicken Cold Noodles
- **Snack**: Honeydew & Cottage Cheese Cup
- **Dinner**: Tofu Stir-Fry with Veggies

Day 27
- **Breakfast**: Coconut & Blueberry Chia Pudding with a side of Cinnamon Rice Cereal Delight
- **Lunch**: Cannellini Bean and Carrot Soup with a side of Broccoli & Quinoa Bowl
- **Snack**: Seed Crackers with Avocado Dip
- **Dinner**: Lemon-Poached Cod with Spinach

Day 28
- **Breakfast**: Buckwheat & Berry Bowl with a side of Whole Grain Pancakes
- **Lunch**: Zucchini Noodles with Pesto with a side of Spinach, Quinoa, and Avocado Salad
- **Snack**: Edamame & Sea Salt
- **Dinner**: Eggplant & Chickpea Curry

Day 29
- **Breakfast**: Oatmeal with Apple and Chia Seeds with a side of Greens Morning Juice
- **Lunch**: Zucchini Noodles with Pesto with a side of Steamed Sea Bass Fillet with Fennel
- **Snack**: Sunflower Seed & Date Balls
- **Dinner**: Tofu Stir-Fry with Veggies

Day 30
- **Breakfast**: Refined-Sugar-Free Apple & Cinnamon Crepes with a side of Mint & Melon Medley
- **Lunch**: Cannellini Bean and Carrot Soup with a side of Rice Pilaf with Almonds
- **Snack**: Carrot & Cucumber Pinwheels
- **Dinner**: Butternut & Barley Risotto

Day 31
- **Breakfast**: Whole Grain Pancakes with a side of Blueberry and Almond Milk Smoothie
- **Lunch**: Tuna & Avocado Salad with a side of Broccoli & Quinoa Bowl
- **Snack**: Date & Walnut Energy Bites
- **Dinner**: Grilled Tilapia with Herbed Quinoa

Day 32
- **Breakfast**: Banana & Almond Butter Oats with a side of Soothing Ginger-Pear Smoothie
- **Lunch**: Rustic Root Vegetable Medley with a side of Silky Sesame & Chicken Cold Noodles
- **Snack**: Mango Rice Cakes
- **Dinner**: Baked Quinoa and Spinach Patties

Day 33
- **Breakfast**: Omega-Rich Chia & Hemp Seed Parfait with a side of Whole Grain Pancakes
- **Lunch**: Polenta with Sautéed Greens with a side of Golden Beet & Barley Bowl with Lemon Zest
- **Snack**: Lemon-Mint Yogurt Pops
- **Dinner**: Quinoa and Roasted Root Vegetable Salad

Day 34
- **Breakfast**: Coconut & Blueberry Chia Pudding with a side of Flaxseed Morning Muffins
- **Lunch**: Pea & Mint Risotto with a side of Roasted Vegetable Platter
- **Snack**: Coconut and Sunflower Seed Energy Bars
- **Dinner**: Fennel & White Bean Stew

Day 35
- **Breakfast**: Avocado Toast on Sprouted Bread with a side of Cinnamon Rice Cereal Delight
- **Lunch**: Steamed Sea Bass Fillet with Fennel with a side of Zucchini Noodles with Pesto
- **Snack**: Seed Crackers with Avocado Dip
- **Dinner**: Lemon-Poached Cod with Spinach

Day 36
- **Breakfast**: Golden Turmeric Oatmeal with a side of Fresh Greens Morning Juice
- **Lunch**: Broccoli & Quinoa Bowl with a side of Eggplant & Chickpea Curry
- **Snack**: Sunflower Seed & Date Balls
- **Dinner**: Grilled Tilapia with Herbed Quinoa

Day 37
- **Breakfast**: Soothing Ginger-Pear Smoothie with a side of Omega-Rich Chia & Hemp Seed Parfait
- **Lunch**: Spinach, Quinoa, and Avocado Salad with a side of Silky Sesame & Chicken Cold Noodles
- **Snack**: Toasted Almond & Raisin Mix
- **Dinner**: Savory Stuffed Acorn Squash

Day 38

- **Breakfast**: Banana & Almond Butter Oats with a side of Coconut & Blueberry Chia Pudding
- **Lunch**: Zucchini Noodles with Pesto with a side of Cannellini Bean and Carrot Soup
- **Snack**: Carrot & Cucumber Pinwheels
- **Dinner**: Mushroom & Brown Rice Bowl

Day 39

- **Breakfast**: Avocado Toast on Sprouted Bread with a side of Mint & Melon Medley
- **Lunch**: Pea & Mint Risotto with a side of Polenta with Sautéed Greens
- **Snack**: Lemon-Mint Yogurt Pops
- **Dinner**: Tofu Stir-Fry with Veggies

Day 40

- **Breakfast**: Flaxseed Morning Muffins with a side of Soothing Ginger-Pear Smoothie
- **Lunch**: Steamed Sea Bass Fillet with Fennel with a side of Golden Beet & Barley Bowl with Lemon Zest
- **Snack**: Coconut and Sunflower Seed Energy Bars
- **Dinner**: Baked Quinoa and Spinach Patties

Day 41

- **Breakfast**: Cinnamon Rice Cereal Delight with a side of Whole Grain Pancakes
- **Lunch**: Tuna & Avocado Salad with a side of Broccoli & Quinoa Bowl
- **Snack**: Seed Crackers with Avocado Dip
- **Dinner**: Fennel & White Bean Stew

Day 42

- **Breakfast**: Buckwheat & Berry Bowl with a side of Coconut & Blueberry Chia Pudding
- **Lunch**: Rustic Root Vegetable Medley with a side of Silky Sesame & Chicken Cold Noodles
- **Snack**: Date & Walnut Energy Bites
- **Dinner**: Quinoa and Roasted Root Vegetable Salad

Day 43

- **Breakfast**: Refined-Sugar-Free Apple & Cinnamon Crepes with a side of Golden Turmeric Oatmeal
- **Lunch**: Broccoli & Quinoa Bowl with a side of Roasted Vegetable Platter
- **Snack**: Mango Rice Cakes
- **Dinner**: Grilled Tilapia with Herbed Quinoa

Day 44

- **Breakfast**: Tofu & Spinach Breakfast Scramble with a side of Greens Morning Juice
- **Lunch**: Polenta with Sautéed Greens with a side of Steamed Sea Bass Fillet with Fennel
- **Snack**: Sunflower Seed & Date Balls
- **Dinner**: Mushroom & Brown Rice Bowl

Day 45

- **Breakfast**: Avocado Toast on Sprouted Bread with a side of Banana & Almond Butter Oats
- **Lunch**: Cannellini Bean and Carrot Soup with a side of Zucchini Noodles with Pesto
- **Snack**: Coconut and Sunflower Seed Energy Bars
- **Dinner**: Eggplant & Chickpea Curry

Day 46
- **Breakfast**: Coconut & Blueberry Chia Pudding with a side of Flaxseed Morning Muffins
- **Lunch**: Tuna & Avocado Salad with a side of Rice Pilaf with Almonds
- **Snack**: Lemon-Mint Yogurt Pops
- **Dinner**: Quinoa and Roasted Root Vegetable Salad

Day 47
- **Breakfast**: Omega-Rich Chia & Hemp Seed Parfait with a side of Soothing Ginger-Pear Smoothie
- **Lunch**: Silky Sesame & Chicken Cold Noodles with a side of Broccoli & Quinoa Bowl
- **Snack**: Carrot & Cucumber Pinwheels
- **Dinner**: Fennel & White Bean Stew

Day 48
- **Breakfast**: Whole Grain Pancakes with a side of Mint & Melon Medley
- **Lunch**: Golden Beet & Barley Bowl with Lemon Zest with a side of Spinach, Quinoa, and Avocado Salad
- **Snack**: Date & Walnut Energy Bites
- **Dinner**: Tofu Stir-Fry with Veggies

Day 49
- **Breakfast**: Buckwheat & Berry Bowl with a side of Cinnamon Rice Cereal Delight
- **Lunch**: Rustic Root Vegetable Medley with a side of Cannellini Bean and Carrot Soup
- **Snack**: Edamame & Sea Salt
- **Dinner**: Baked Quinoa and Spinach Patties

Day 50
- **Breakfast**: Golden Turmeric Oatmeal with a side of Cucumber and Zucchini Smoothie
- **Lunch**: Broccoli & Quinoa Bowl with a side of Polenta with Sautéed Greens
- **Snack**: Toasted Oats & Banana Bars
- **Dinner**: Baked Falafel with Tzatziki

Day 51
- **Breakfast**: Avocado Toast on Sprouted Bread with a side of Soothing Ginger-Pear Smoothie
- **Lunch**: Steamed Sea Bass Fillet with Fennel with a side of Zucchini Noodles with Pesto
- **Snack**: Coconut and Sunflower Seed Energy Bars
- **Dinner**: Tofu Stir-Fry with Veggies

Day 52
- **Breakfast**: Banana & Almond Butter Oats with a side of Coconut & Blueberry Chia Pudding
- **Lunch**: Tuna & Avocado Salad with a side of Golden Beet & Barley Bowl with Lemon Zest
- **Snack**: Carrot & Cucumber Pinwheels
- **Dinner**: Butternut & Barley Risotto

Day 53
- **Breakfast**: Omega-Rich Chia & Hemp Seed Parfait with a side of Refined-Sugar-Free Apple & Cinnamon Crepes
- **Lunch**: Silky Sesame & Chicken Cold Noodles with a side of Roasted Vegetable Platter
- **Snack**: Date & Walnut Energy Bites
- **Dinner**: Quinoa and Roasted Root Vegetable Salad

Day 54

- **Breakfast**: Flaxseed Morning Muffins with a side of Greens Morning Juice
- **Lunch**: Spinach, Quinoa, and Avocado Salad with a side of Cannellini Bean and Carrot Soup
- **Snack**: Lemon-Mint Yogurt Pops
- **Dinner**: Eggplant & Chickpea Curry

Day 55

- **Breakfast**: Cinnamon Rice Cereal Delight with a side of Banana & Almond Butter Oats
- **Lunch**: Broccoli & Quinoa Bowl with a side of Pea & Mint Risotto
- **Snack**: Mango Rice Cakes
- **Dinner**: Fennel & White Bean Stew

Day 56

- **Breakfast**: Coconut & Blueberry Chia Pudding with a side of Whole Grain Pancakes
- **Lunch**: Rustic Root Vegetable Medley with a side of Tuna & Avocado Salad
- **Snack**: Sunflower Seed & Date Balls
- **Dinner**: Lemon-Poached Cod with Spinach

Day 57

- **Breakfast**: Whole Grain Pancakes with a side of Soothing Ginger-Pear Smoothie
- **Lunch**: Golden Beet & Barley Bowl with Lemon Zest with a side of Steamed Sea Bass Fillet with Fennel
- **Snack**: Carrot & Cucumber Pinwheels
- **Dinner**: Tofu Stir-Fry with Veggies

Day 58

- **Breakfast**: Banana & Almond Butter Oats with a side of Coconut & Blueberry Chia Pudding
- **Lunch**: Polenta with Sautéed Greens with a side of Spinach, Quinoa, and Avocado Salad
- **Snack**: Coconut and Sunflower Seed Energy Bars
- **Dinner**: Savory Stuffed Acorn Squash

Day 59

- **Breakfast**: Avocado Toast on Sprouted Bread with a side of Greens Morning Juice
- **Lunch**: Cannellini Bean and Carrot Soup with a side of Silky Sesame & Chicken Cold Noodles
- **Snack**: Date & Walnut Energy Bites
- **Dinner**: Baked Quinoa and Spinach Patties

Day 60

- **Breakfast**: Omega-Rich Chia & Hemp Seed Parfait with a side of Flaxseed Morning Muffins
- **Lunch**: Tuna & Avocado Salad with a side of Broccoli & Quinoa Bowl
- **Snack**: Honeydew & Cottage Cheese Cup
- **Dinner**: Fennel & White Bean Stew

Chapter 10: Beyond food: lifestyle tweaks

Altering daily habits for profound relief

Let's talk about how we can elevate our day-to-day routines to not only manage acid reflux but also to amplify our overall well-being. It's more than just what we eat; it's how we eat, how we move, and even how we dress and rest.

First and foremost, have you ever considered the timing of your meals? Starting your day with a balanced breakfast isn't just a cliché – it really sets the digestive mood for the entire day. And while we're on the subject of time, try to wrap up your dinner a few hours before hitting the bed. This gives your stomach a breather and prevents those pesky nighttime reflux episodes. Also, think about the size of your meals. Instead of feasting on three big meals, how about five smaller ones? It's like giving your stomach bite-sized tasks instead of overwhelming projects.

When you do sit down for a meal, make it a point to be present. Chew your food slowly, relish every bite. It's not just about savoring the flavor, but it also aids digestion and helps you understand when you're full.

After meals, resist that urge to slump on the couch or dive into bed. Give gravity a chance to help out. An upright posture keeps that stomach acid in check, and if you're up for it, a gentle post-meal stroll can be a game-changer.

While we're discussing changes, think about your weight. Every little pound can make a difference. A bit of extra weight, especially around your middle, can make reflux more frequent. So, staying active not only gets you in shape but also promotes smoother digestion.

Water, as they say, is life. Keep yourself hydrated. Just remember to slow down on the liquids during meals. And if you're a caffeine enthusiast, maybe cut back a little – your stomach will thank you.

Now, here's a simple tip that many overlook: your clothing choice. Tight belts and constricting waistbands? Maybe save them for those special occasions. On regular days, give priority to comfort.

Sleeping with an elevated head can be a game-changer. It's simple physics, really. By lifting your head a few inches, you make it harder for the acid to creep up. There are even pillows designed for this!

Let's also touch upon the importance of a calm mind. Stress can rile up your gut. So, breathe deep, try meditation, or maybe dabble in yoga. Setting aside a bit of "you" time can have wonderful effects on your digestion and overall well-being.

Lastly, if you're a smoker or enjoy your alcoholic beverages, it might be time for some reflection. Smoking can make reflux more common, and excessive alcohol doesn't do your stomach lining any favors.

Mindful eating and the benefits of paced consumption

In today's hustle and bustle, isn't it peculiar that eating, one of life's most essential and delightful experiences, is often rushed? Dive into the world of mindful eating with me and let's explore the beauty and benefits of truly savoring our meals.

So, you might be wondering, what exactly is mindful eating? Think of it as an immersive experience. It's not just about wolfing down your food, but truly being in the moment with every bite you take. It's an age-old concept, inspired by Buddhist teachings, where the act of eating becomes a meditative experience.

Now, when we eat in haste, it's not just our palate that's missing out. Our stomach isn't a fan either. Rushing through our meals can lead to all sorts of digestive upsets, including that pesky acid reflux. And, without even realizing it, we might end up consuming more than we need, which is not too friendly for our waistlines either.

Let's pivot to paced consumption. Picture this: a mealtime free from distractions. No screens, no buzzing notifications, just you and your food. Make each bite count. Give it a good 20 to 30 chews, letting yourself appreciate its taste and texture. Then, take a moment. Breathe. Enjoy the flavor and then proceed.

What does this do for you? First off, your digestion thanks you. It's easier to break down well-chewed food, ensuring you get all those vital nutrients. Being in sync with your body's signals can help keep those extra pounds at bay. Moreover, by truly engaging with your food, you heighten the joy of eating. And here's a bonus: a calmer, slower approach to eating can keep those acid reflux flare-ups in check. Plus, it's like a mini-meditation session. Your mind gets a break, and often, a calmer mind equates to a happier gut.

Starting this journey can feel overwhelming. So, here are a few nudges in the right direction. Begin your meals with a silent 'thank you' for the nourishment on your plate. Be it a full-course meal or a simple snack, eat with all your senses engaged. And every so often, check in with yourself. Are you still hungry or just eating out of habit? Remember, even when you're dining out or amidst friends, take a moment to relish your meal.

Like all good things, mastering mindful eating does take time. There might be days when old habits creep in. It's okay. Gently remind yourself to come back to the moment. Keeping a journal might help. Pen down your experiences, the highs and lows, and soon, you'll see patterns and understand your relationship with food better.

Portion sizes and optimal meal frequencies

Ever wondered if there's more to managing digestive health than just selecting the right foods? Let's dive deep into the world of portion control and the significance of meal frequencies.

First, let's talk about the portion sizes. Eating more than your body needs is like filling a car with excess fuel; it's unnecessary and can lead to problems. Not only does it strain our digestion, but it also often results in that all-too-familiar feeling of being overstuffed. Plus, keeping portions in check is a trusted ally in maintaining our weight. Wondering how to gauge the right amount? Think of familiar objects for reference, like visualizing a serving of meat as the size of a deck of cards. And yes, those nutrition labels on food packages? They're goldmines of information. Equip yourself with measuring tools like cups and spoons or simply use smaller plates. Remember, it's not about eating less, but eating right.

Now, let's venture into meal frequencies. While many of us grew up with the conventional three meals a day, some find that smaller meals spread throughout the day can be kinder to their stomachs. This is especially true for those prone to reflux. But here's the golden rule: Listen to your body. It's the most reliable guide you'll ever have. Consistency is crucial; setting a regular eating schedule can help your body find its rhythm. And if you're snacking in between, make those snacks count nutritionally. One more thing, aim to wrap up your meals a few hours before you hit the sack. It helps keep nighttime reflux at bay.

Stepping out for a meal? Keep in mind, restaurants tend to be quite generous with their portions. Splitting dishes or packing up leftovers is perfectly alright. And at social gatherings, it's okay to politely decline that extra serving. Let's also address the elephant in the room: emotional eating. It's essential to understand what drives us to overeat, whether it's stress, sadness, or sheer boredom.

So, what's in it for you if you master portion control and meal timing? A more comfortable digestive system, for starters. Steady energy levels, a check on weight, and a healthier relationship with food.

Chapter 11: Reflux FAQs & tips for the real world

Decoding common queries about acid reflux and food choices

The interplay between diet and acid reflux is a topic of intrigue for many, leading to a plethora of questions that revolve around food choices, meal timings, and nutritional strategies. This chapter is dedicated to answering some of the most frequently asked questions, providing clarity and practical advice to guide readers on their reflux management journey.

1. Can I ever eat my favorite trigger foods again?

- **The Concept of Moderation**: How some might reintroduce problematic foods gradually and in smaller quantities.
- **Personal Variation**: Understanding that reactions to trigger foods can differ from person to person and might change over time.

2. Are spicy foods universally bad for acid reflux?

- **Differing Tolerance Levels**: While spicy foods can be a trigger for many, some individuals may tolerate them better.
- **Test and Trial**: Methods to gauge personal reactions to different levels of spice.

3. Is it true that smaller, more frequent meals can help manage reflux?

- **Benefits of Portion Control**: Explaining how smaller meals can reduce stomach pressure and minimize reflux episodes.
- **Balancing Nutrient Intake**: Ensuring adequate nutrition even when consuming smaller quantities.

4. Does drinking water with meals exacerbate symptoms?

- **Hydration and Digestion**: Understanding how water can aid digestion but also potentially dilute stomach acid.
- **Finding Your Balance**: Tips to optimize water intake during meals without exacerbating symptoms.

5. Are there any natural remedies that can soothe acid reflux?

- **Herbal Teas and Infusions**: The potential benefits of chamomile, ginger, and other herbal teas.
- **Aloe Vera and Slippery Elm**: Exploring their roles in soothing the digestive tract.

6. Does laying down after a meal increase the chances of reflux?

- **Gravity and Digestion**: How a reclining position can allow acid to flow back into the esophagus more easily.
- **Optimal Post-Meal Activities**: Suggestions on how to minimize reflux occurrences after eating.

7. Can probiotics help with acid reflux?

- **Gut Health and Reflux**: The potential link between a healthy gut microbiome and reduced reflux symptoms.
- **Choosing the Right Probiotic**: Guidance on selecting and consuming probiotic supplements.

8. Is caffeine a no-go for reflux sufferers?

- **Caffeine and LES Relaxation**: How caffeine can potentially weaken the lower esophageal sphincter, leading to acid reflux.
- **Moderation and Alternatives**: Exploring reduced caffeine intake and alternatives like herbal teas.

9. How does alcohol impact acid reflux?

- **Alcohol and Stomach Acid**: Understanding how alcohol can increase stomach acid production.
- **Making Informed Choices**: Tips on selecting drinks that are less likely to trigger reflux and practicing moderation.

10. Are there specific cooking methods better suited for acid reflux sufferers?

- **The Merits of Steaming and Grilling**: Exploring gentler cooking methods that preserve nutrient integrity and are less likely to exacerbate reflux.
- **Foods to Avoid Frying**: Guidance on which foods can become more reflux-inducing when fried.

Overcoming everyday challenges of living with reflux

Living with acid reflux isn't just about the physical discomfort; it's also about navigating the social, emotional, and lifestyle challenges that arise. From dining out with friends to traveling or handling stress, managing reflux requires an awareness of its triggers and strategies to minimize flare-ups. This chapter offers actionable insights to handle these challenges with grace and confidence.

1. Dining Out and Social Events

- **Reading Between the Menu Lines**: Tips for identifying and selecting reflux-friendly options at restaurants.
- **Open Communication**: Importance of voicing dietary preferences and limitations to hosts or servers.
- **Alcohol Alternatives**: Suggesting non-alcoholic beverages that won't trigger reflux during social gatherings.

2. Traveling with Acid Reflux

- **Packing the Essentials**: Creating a travel kit with antacids, prescribed medications, and other essentials.
- **Navigating Airplane Meals**: Making informed choices when flying.
- **Staying Prepared Abroad**: Tips for researching and finding reflux-friendly foods in foreign countries.

3. Managing Stress and Anxiety

- **Mind-Body Connection**: Understanding how stress can exacerbate reflux symptoms.
- **Relaxation Techniques**: Introducing methods like meditation, deep breathing, and progressive muscle relaxation.
- **Seeking Support**: Recognizing when it's beneficial to consult a therapist or counselor.

4. Balancing Work and Reflux

- **Meal Prepping for the Office**: Strategies for preparing and packing reflux-friendly lunches.
- **Handling Business Dinners**: Tips for navigating work-related dining events without triggering symptoms.

- **Incorporating Breaks**: The importance of taking short breaks to manage stress and facilitate digestion.

5. Sleep Strategies for Reflux Sufferers

- **Optimal Sleep Positions**: Discussing how elevating the head and sleeping on the left side can reduce nighttime reflux.
- **Creating a Pre-Bed Routine**: Emphasizing the importance of avoiding heavy meals and certain activities before sleep.

6. Navigating Fitness and Exercise

- **Exercise Selection**: Understanding which exercises can help or hinder reflux symptoms.
- **Timing it Right**: Recommendations on the best times to exercise in relation to meals.
- **Staying Hydrated**: Tips for drinking water during workouts without triggering reflux.

7. Pregnancy and Acid Reflux

- **Hormonal Impact**: Discussing how pregnancy hormones can affect reflux.
- **Safe Management Strategies**: Offering guidance on managing reflux during pregnancy while ensuring the safety of both mother and baby.

8. Handling Comments and Misconceptions

- **Educating Loved Ones**: Providing ways to explain acid reflux to friends and family who might not understand.
- **Building Resilience**: Tips for dealing with unsolicited advice or comments without getting discouraged.

9. Celebrations, Holidays, and Festive Feasts

- **Anticipating Triggers**: Preparing for potential triggers during festive meals.
- **Making Reflux-Friendly Alternatives**: Recipes and ideas for creating delicious, festive foods that won't cause discomfort.

Navigating restaurant menus and social dining gracefully

Dining out should be a pleasurable experience, a blend of culinary exploration and social bonding. However, for those with acid reflux, restaurant menus can seem like minefields. This chapter delves into strategies to enjoy dining out without triggering an episode, ensuring that the joy of shared meals remains undiminished.

1. Research in Advance

- **The Power of Preparation**: Why doing a little homework before heading to a restaurant can help in making informed choices.
- **Checking Menus Online**: The advantage of previewing menu items and identifying potential safe options.

2. Open Dialogue with Restaurant Staff

- **Effective Communication**: The importance of talking to servers or chefs about your dietary restrictions.
- **Asking the Right Questions**: Key questions to ask about meal ingredients, preparation methods, and potential substitutions.

3. Recognizing Common Culprits on Menus

- **Stealthy Triggers**: Identifying foods that may seem innocent but can exacerbate reflux.
- **Decoding Menu Jargon**: Translating common culinary terms that may indicate reflux-triggering preparation methods.

4. Alcohol and Beverages

- **Choosing Wisely**: Suggesting beverages that are less likely to trigger reflux.
- **Alternatives to Alcohol**: Non-alcoholic drink options that are both delicious and reflux-friendly.

5. Appetizers and Starters

- **Safe Bets**: Recommending appetizers that are typically gentle on the stomach.
- **Avoiding the Pitfalls**: Highlighting popular starters that might trigger acid reflux and suggesting alternatives.

6. Main Courses

- **Grilled Over Fried**: Emphasizing the benefits of opting for grilled, steamed, or roasted dishes.
- **Sauce Savvy**: Understanding and navigating sauces that might be too rich or acidic.

7. Desserts

- **Sweet without the Burn**: Identifying desserts that are less likely to cause discomfort.
- **Moderation is Key**: Enjoying treats in smaller portions to avoid overwhelming the stomach.

8. Buffets and Multi-Course Meals

- **Pacing Yourself**: The benefits of slow and mindful eating, especially when faced with an abundance of choices.
- **Strategic Selection**: Navigating buffets by scanning all options first and then making informed choices.

9. Social Dining Etiquette

- **Declining Gracefully**: How to politely refuse food without offending the host or drawing undue attention.
- **Educating Curious Minds**: Handling questions about dietary restrictions with poise.

10. Handling Unexpected Reflux Episodes

- **Staying Calm**: Strategies for managing sudden discomfort in public.
- **Emergency Kit**: Keeping a small kit with antacids or prescribed medications when dining out.

Conclusion

Let's dive into a reflective chat about the journey with acid reflux you've walked through.

So, you've come a long way, haven't you? Remember those early days, when understanding and grappling with reflux felt like an uphill battle? Now, think about the positive changes you've made in your diet, the habits you've nurtured, and how you've managed to ease some of those symptoms. That's commendable growth and progress.

Listening to your body has been pivotal. It's like tuning into a radio frequency, catching signals, and understanding its messages. That symptom diary you've been keeping? A real game-changer. It's helped in making some informed choices. However, it's essential to remember that our bodies aren't static. They change, and so does their reaction to certain foods. But that's okay. Life's all about adapting, right? It's about periodically revisiting our diet and lifestyle choices and tweaking them if necessary.

On this journey, have you connected with others facing similar challenges? There's comfort in knowing you're not alone, and there's so much to learn from shared experiences. It's a tight-knit community of reflux warriors!

Beyond the physical symptoms, it's undeniable that living with a chronic condition can be mentally and emotionally taxing. But remember, self-love is paramount. Embrace yourself, imperfections and all. Mental well-being is just as vital in this healing journey. Staying informed about the latest research on acid reflux is beneficial. Also, why not use your journey to help others? Sharing your experiences can be a beacon of light for someone just starting out.

So, what's next? Maybe you're thinking of trying out a new reflux-friendly recipe or perhaps exploring a relaxation technique? Envision a future where reflux is better managed, and set tangible milestones to reach that vision.

Setbacks? They're a part of the journey. Some days might be tougher than others, but they don't define your entire story. Whenever there's a stumble, gather your tools, and techniques and get back on track.

Life with acid reflux is about more than just symptom management. It's about experiencing a wholesome life despite the challenges. With all you've learned and the community you've found, the future looks bright. So, move forward with hope, resilience, and the comforting thought that you're never journeying solo.

Now, onto an uplifting note.

Life with acid reflux often feels like a never-ending cycle of discomfort and constant dietary shifts. Yet, there's a silver lining. Living this reflux-conscious life has probably made you more mindful of your overall health and even sparked culinary adventures. And remember, every challenge faced only adds to your resilience.

Celebrate the small wins. Perhaps it's a day with lesser discomfort, or maybe you found a delicious meal that didn't trigger any symptoms. These moments? They're building your confidence.

Outside the realm of diet, maybe you've discovered new hobbies or revisited old ones, finding solace and joy in art, travel, or even literature. Have you shared your story? Your journey can be an inspiration for many, showing them they aren't alone. And in return, their stories might uplift you. Even amidst the discomfort, there are countless moments of joy – a peaceful walk, time with loved ones, or just losing yourself in a beautiful melody. These moments, they're the ones that make memories. A holistic approach to well-being is beneficial. While diet plays a role, focusing on mental, emotional, and even spiritual well-being can provide a comprehensive healing touch.

The future? It holds promise. Stay optimistic about medical advancements and envision a life where reflux is just a part, not your entire tale.

Remember, while acid reflux is a chapter in your life, it isn't your whole story. Ahead are unwritten pages brimming with adventures, happiness, lessons, and resilience tales. Approach them with an open heart, knowing that the best is yet to come.

CREDITS

Image by <a
href="https://www.freepik.com/free-photo/flat-lay-pancakes-with-mix-fruits_6037924.htm#query=Heartburn-Free%20Whole%20Grain%20Pancakes
&position=12&from_view=search&track=ais&uuid=02db55fb-9f75-40c6-8d37-7c834fffe788">Freepik</a>
Image by <a
href="https://www.freepik.com/free-photo/pasta-with-green-herbs_1807936.htm#query=Whole%20Grain%20Pasta%20with%20Olive%20Oil%20Dri
zzle&position=20&from_view=search&track=ais&uuid=ca18b142-c14b-4538-9e04-64db026e0714">Freepik</a>
<a
href="https://www.freepik.com/free-photo/salad-with-cucumber-couscous-feta_28007142.htm#query=Nutty%20Bulgur%20and%20Veggie%20Salad
%20feta%20almond&position=0&from_view=search&track=ais&uuid=3435f2e2-72ff-4366-9301-b117944feeea">Image by fahrwasser</a> on
Freepik
<a
href="https://www.freepik.com/free-photo/tasty-appetizing-crispbread-with-mashed-avocado-served-plate_15772946.htm#query=Crackers%20Salti
ne%20Spread%20with%20Avocado&position=2&from_view=search&track=ais&uuid=93daf942-8442-466c-909e-706d6336eedd">Image by
valeria_aksakova</a> on Freepik
Image by <a
href="https://www.freepik.com/free-photo/immunity-boosting-foods-healthy-life_21076846.htm#query=Green%20Ginger%20Tea&position=0&from_
view=search&track=ais&uuid=6584bf9e-d45a-49b9-8789-3cd6ee96ec73">Freepik</a>
<a
href="https://www.freepik.com/free-photo/pilaf-with-vegetables-greens_7722779.htm#fromView=search&page=1&position=31&uuid=2ea93198-b93
a-49f1-8fb9-31e17e669951">Image by cookie_studio on Freepik</a>
<a
href="https://www.freepik.com/free-photo/shawarma-from-juicy-beef-lettuce-tomatoes-cucumbers-paprika-onion-pita-bread-with-spinach-diet-menu_
7122681.htm#fromView=search&page=1&position=3&uuid=21c40089-4e15-48f1-a3b9-05c6d517b581">Image by timolina on Freepik</a>

SCAN THE QR-CODE

Made in the USA
Monee, IL
05 November 2024

69178641R00063